THE **MEN'S HEALTH** BOOK

A Guide for the Irish Man

DR MARK ROWE

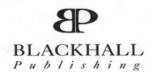
BP
BLACKHALL
Publishing

Blackhall Publishing
Lonsdale House
Avoca Avenue
Blackrock
Co. Dublin
Ireland

e-mail: info@blackhallpublishing.com
www.blackhallpublishing.com

ISBN: 978-1-84218-165-2

A catalogue record for this book is available from the British Library.

Printed in Ireland by ColourBooks Ltd.

I dedicate this book to Edel and our children
Malcolm, Tony and Lydia.

I also dedicate it to my late father, Brendan Rowe,
who inspired me to write it.

Finally, I dedicate this book to the many heroes out there who work
hard on a daily basis to make a difference to the lives of others.

Dr Mark Rowe – Biographical Information

Mark Rowe is a General Practitioner with a special interest in men's health. He graduated from UCD Medical School in 1991 and went on to specialise in family practice and became a qualified member of the Irish College of General Practitioners in 1995, achieving the first place 'Ellerd Eppel' award. Since then he has practised as a GP in Waterford City. He also runs a men's health programme at the Waterford Health Park where his practice is based.

He is a trainer with the South-East GP Training Programme. He is also an examiner with the Irish College of General Practitioners. Dr Rowe has published a number of national guidelines and articles in the Irish College of General Practitioners' journal, *Forum*.

He has given seminars and has acted as guest speaker on the topic of men's health at a number of events.

He ran the New York Marathon in 2007 and fundraised for two charities. His current research interest is in the area of 'generative space', which means that by providing inspiring surroundings in the primary healthcare setting you can enhance the esteem and feel-good factor of both patients and staff, with resultant long-term health improvements.

Acknowledgements

It is with deep gratitude that I express my appreciation to the following for their contributions to the *Men's Health Book*:

- To my patients, whom I am privileged to serve on a daily basis. Also to my colleagues and staff, who assist in that care.
- To all the team at Blackhall Publishing: to Elizabeth Brennan for her initial encouragement and to Eileen O'Brien, who reviewed the chapters, set deadlines and suggested improvements.
- To Richard Murphy for his creativity, which is evident in the illustrations throughout the book.
- Finally, to my dear wife Edel, for her help, support and encouragement in this, as in all things.

Contents

Health is the crown on a well man's head that only the sick man can see.

— Anonymous

Preface

We live in the rapidly moving information age, with the latest news, traffic, weather and sport only a finger-tip or text message away. The same applies to information on health, yet, as the saying goes, you can take a horse to water, but you can't make him drink.

As a family doctor with a special interest in men's health. I am aware of the large gap that exists in many cases between Irish men and good health. Indeed, this gap is widening all the time with more and more men succumbing to largely preventable illnesses, often with tragic consequences.

Hence the idea for this book, the aim of which is to simply help bridge the gap in knowledge that sometimes exists on the ground, as well as challenge the prevailing attitudes to healthcare among Irish men. As a family doctor working in a busy city practice I am well aware of the natural reluctance of many Irish men to access healthcare, except in an emergency. Of course none of the information in this book is designed to replace the one-to-one relationship with your doctor. However, I also know from experience that many Irish men don't have a doctor, or at least one they know well enough!

For the Irish man who takes the time and effort to read any, part, or all of this book, I hope it will help give you the confidence to approach your family doctor if and when necessary. I also hope you will understand better the importance of proactively managing your health, just as you would service your own car. The important message is that you can take control of your health and improve it significantly. Prevention is, after all, much better than cure. As they say, a stitch in time saves nine.

Of course men's health affects all of us, not just men. For the women who have fathers, brothers, sons, partners or friends, men's health issues are important for you too. As men we have a responsibility to nurture that gift of good health and to keep ourselves well. This means we need to be willing to change, to accept help, to re-adjust the speedometer and to get a regular service too.

This book is in many ways the product of the current knowledge, thinking and understanding in healthcare of men's health issues. In this regard I am grateful for and wish to acknowledge my medical colleagues worldwide, whose wisdom, experience and research has brought medicine to where it is today. And still the journey of exploration continues. The one certainty in healthcare is that the only constant is change. This means that new, pioneering breakthroughs can become established best practice and replace existing treatments. But the foundations of good health, including a healthy diet and lifestyle with plenty of exercise, remain constant. The more things change, the more they stay the same.

As a doctor I can appreciate every day just how wonderful the gift of good health is. All parents have a tremendous opportunity to help nurture their children, who will become the men and women of tomorrow. Leading by example can help children to model their behaviour on ours so that healthy habits learned young can be engrained for ever. This applies to exercise, diet and a whole range of physical and mental health and lifestyle issues.

I hope that this book will give men the knowledge, confidence and courage to take control of their own health and not become another statistic. Men owe this to the mothers who reared them, to the partners who take care of and worry about them and to the children who depend on them. But, most importantly of all, men owe it to themselves.

I hope this book will make a difference.

All royalties from this book will go to the men's cancer division of the Marie Keating Foundation, who work passionately and tirelessly to promote men's cancer awareness.

1

The Health Hazards of Being Male

007 – A Real Man's Hero

In the movies, James Bond is the quintessential bulletproof male. He just doesn't 'do' healthcare. He gets shot at, ambushed, beaten up regularly and still keeps coming back for more. 'Shaken, not stirred', as the saying goes. He perceives himself to be pretty much invincible. He can sail off into the sunset after every life-threatening encounter, battered and bruised but always ready for the next round of double martinis.

Real-life stories are rather different, however. Many Irish men think their health is 'excellent' – and they're literally dying on their feet to prove it. Irish men live shorter lives than Irish women and have a higher risk of serious illness. Compared to women, men are often less interested in and less knowledgeable about health matters and are less likely to accept personal responsibility for their health. These health beliefs of men are linked with behaviour that hinders their health and an increased risk of death and disease.

This tendency to not go to the doctor combines with lifestyle behaviour often best left to Hollywood stuntmen. The result is a shortened lifespan; by about five to six years on average compared to women. Men perceive themselves as being less susceptible to ill health than women. This is a false and dangerous assumption, which further increases their health risks. Many men fail to get routine check-ups, preventative care or health counselling. They often ignore symptoms or delay seeking medical attention when sick or in pain.

There is no doubt about it, being male is a health hazard.

Men are from Mars, Women are from Venus

It is clear that the two sexes are different, not just in the obvious bio-logical ways, but in every system of their bodies. Far from being the stronger sex, we men are more fragile throughout our lives. This male fragility can be partly explained by the different ways in which men and women approach health, healthcare and illness. Men are less likely to discuss health and personal issues with friends than women are and they are also less likely to access healthcare services. Unfortunately, men often suffer in silence, disregarding the symp-toms of a potentially serious condition, to their cost. There may be many factors that help to predetermine the shorter lifespan for men in comparison to women.

Lack of Knowledge

Men tend to have poorer knowledge of basic health information and less understanding of the anatomy and functions of their own bod-ies than women. This knowledge gap in the basic anatomy of the human body makes some men embarrassed to seek health advice. Most men know more about how the home heating system works or the internal mechanics of their car than they know about the sys-tems at work in their own bodies. Indeed, women may have a better understanding of the male body than many men have themselves. As a result:

- Many men will not attend the doctor unless told to do so by their partner, and admit to waiting too long before seeing their doctor with a worrying health issue.
- Many men do not know what the prostate gland does or where it is located and are not aware of the common symptoms of prostate cancer.
- Many young men are not aware that men under thirty are in the highest risk group for testicular cancer. Only a minority of young men know about and practise testicular self-examination, which is tragic as early detection of this common cancer in young men almost always guarantees cure.
- The majority of men do not acknowledge 21 units of alcohol per week as a safe drinking limit for males.

The Male Genes

Men differ from women in that men have a different genetic make-up. We all have twenty-three pairs of chromosomes. The difference between men and women is in the twenty-third pair, known as the sex chromosomes. We men have a Y chromosome, whereas the fairer sex don't. The presence of this Y chromosome confers our maleness on us, which means we produce testosterone. The male hormone testosterone is believed to be the cause of male aggression. The tendency to aggression can have adverse health consequences, notably resulting in more violence and more accidents. This can lead to more deaths from both road traffic and work-related accidents, as well as more incidence of homicide and suicide in men, particularly young men. Testosterone may also make men more prone to risky behaviour, including casual sexual encounters, use of illicit drugs and binge drinking. All of this risk-taking behaviour can have adverse health consequences.

Hormones

Hormonal differences between men and women may at least partly explain why women live longer than men. Women have lots of oestrogen, the female hormone, and this seems to protect women against heart disease by having beneficial effects on their cholesterol levels, at least until menopause. Men have much less oestrogen in their systems; however, they do have plenty of testosterone. The effects of testosterone on the male system are the subject of ongoing research, but it is thought that it may have adverse effects on cholesterol, encouraging the deposition of fat around the belly area (belly fat), as well as having some effect on the clotting system in the blood.

Testosterone may also have some effects on the ageing process. It is implicated in both benign enlargement of the prostate gland and the development of prostate cancer. Testosterone can also be involved in the development of heart disease and stroke in men.

Doctor Avoidance Syndrome

Men have limited contact with the health services compared to women. Men are often afraid to seek medical help when sick and can struggle to openly acknowledge fear as a normal part of coping with sickness. This fear or anxiety about going to the doctor may relate to the prospect of having private parts examined, concern about having a serious condition diagnosed or fear of having to go to hospital. One of the big challenges for men is to accept that going to the doctor does not represent failure or personal weakness.

Men often go late to the doctor with an illness when symptoms may have been present for some time. This can also be called 'head in the sand' or 'ostrich' syndrome. You would often hear a man say,

'Sure I am as fit as a fiddle. I haven't been to the doctor in over twenty years.' This doctor avoidance mentality has to change and men need to become more proactive about their own health – after all, they will bring the car to be serviced once a year, why not give themselves the same treatment?

Stress and Distress

Women tend to be more in touch with their feelings and to have better and stronger social networks. They can call on their friends to discuss worries and problems. They are generally better able to communicate their feelings, which has a positive de-stressing effect. This strong sense of socialisation is good for your health.

On the other hand, men tend to be less communicative, bottle up their feelings, internalise stress and soldier on regardless. Indeed, men may be taught as boys to adopt the very attitudes and behaviours that kill them as men: 'big boys don't cry!'

The socially isolated male, dealing with things on his own in his 'own way', can be very bad for his own health, causing stress to turn into distress (see Chapter 14), with its attendant risks of depression, anxiety and potential overdependence on alcohol and/or other drugs. Chronic internalisation of stress can also clog up the arteries and raise blood pressure, helping to cause heart attack and stroke.

Irish men may feel that to access healthcare implies weakness, vulnerability and potential loss of the masculine role. It often requires a health crisis, either personally or in a friend or loved one, to act as a wake-up call.

'Type A' Personality

Type A personality includes such traits as negativity, hostility, anxiety and stress. These behavioural traits are more prevalent in men than in women. It has been associated with an increased risk of heart disease. Psychologists have described the Type A personality as the highly driven macho male. The macho male image of strength and invulnerability does us no favours when it comes to healthcare. It must be one of the reasons why we delay seeking help, trivialise potentially serious health concerns, ignore medical advice and have scant regard for the value of preventative health check-ups. Some men still have a fear of being perceived as a hypochondriac if they ask too many health questions. Again, the implication is that interest in or concern about health matters belies weakness. Well, look at the statistics guys: we continue to die five to six years younger than women, so we have an awful lot of catching up to do before we can be accused of being hypochondriacs.

Solo Run

In general, men value their independence and, as such, are often reluctant to seek medical help. Simply admitting to pain strikes at the core of macho thinking for some men; better to be invincible and 'bulletproof' and eventually fall down in a heap than admit to needing help. This stoical 'grin and bear it' attitude is often admired in a sporting context but, let's face it, it's a terrible way to approach your own health.

Health Risks Every Man Should Know About

The vital statistics of Irish men do not make for encouraging reading. The average male can expect to be seriously or chronically ill for up to fifteen years of his life. The most dangerous health risks are outlined here and the table below shows the main causes of death in Irish men.

Heart Disease

This is the number one killer of Irish men and, together with stroke, accounts for about one in three premature deaths in men. Men usually develop heart disease ten to fifteen years before women do; therefore, men are more likely to die from heart disease in the prime of their lives.

Cancer

Cancer numbers are increasing every year, mainly due to the growth in our population. While cancer can affect all ages, it is most prevalent in the over-65s. The rates of prostate and bowel cancer, while already high, are expected to increase by more than 50 per cent by the year 2020.

Testicular Cancer

Testicular cancer is the most common cause of cancer in men aged 15–35. It is almost always completely curable if it is caught in time. So check your testicles regularly as testicular self-examination may literally save your life. Know your balls!

Prostate Cancer

This is a common cancer in men. Be alert to warning signs of prostate problems, such as having difficulty peeing or regularly getting up during the night to use the bathroom.

Other Cancers

Don't ignore symptoms (such as a persistent cough and blood in the urine or faeces) – early treatment increases the chance of a cure.

Depression and Suicide

Depression is common but often remains unrecognised and undiagnosed in Irish men. Up to one in five Irish men may develop depression in their lives. Suicide is one of the leading causes of death in young Irish men.

Obesity

Over 60 per cent of Irish men are overweight or obese. A waist measurement over 40 inches increases your risk of health problems such as diabetes and heart disease. Eat healthily and lose that gut.

Sexually Transmitted Infections

Up to 50 per cent of men with a sexually transmitted infection don't show any symptoms. Use a condom – prevention is better than cure.

Erectile Dysfunction

Erectile dysfunction issues are very common in Irish men and very treatable. Discuss it with your doctor if you have concerns.

Too Little Exercise

Staying fit is the key to good health. Indeed, exercise may well be the greatest pill of all. Unfortunately, many men take little or not enough exercise, with long-term health consequences.

Smoking

Men still smoke more and die more frequently from smoking than women. It increases the risk of heart disease, half a dozen kinds of cancer and many other illnesses, including emphysema and bronchitis. Half of all smokers will die from their habit if they do not stop. Give it up before it gives you up.

Drinking Alcohol

Many men drink more than the recommended limit of 21 units of alcohol per week. Heavy drinking is common among men. In moderation, alcohol can enhance enjoyment and can reduce the risk of heart disease. In excess, it leads to social and psychological distress and physical damage. Less is more!

The Main Causes of Death in Men

- Heart disease
- Cancer
- Stroke
- Unintentional injuries/accidents
- Suicide
- Chronic lung disease
- Diabetes

You will see from the table above that most of these conditions are largely preventable. So the good news is that, by taking active control of your health, you can keep yourself healthier for longer, hopefully right into ripe old age.

Take Action

As men, we often take pride in our cars and have no problem with the notion of having a full service done on the car annually, or at least every 20,000 miles. Some of us may even take time off work to bring the car to the garage and collect it afterwards. The paradox is that we don't treat our bodies with the same respect. Many Irish men appear to have a lack of awareness of the need for preventative check-ups.

Positive lifestyle changes in men can help prevent heart disease, diabetes, stroke and many diseases and cancers. Effective stress management and a positive outlook can help prevent mid-life depression and feelings of emasculation and uselessness. While a need to win can make a man risk his life, it may also provide the incentive to give up smoking. In fact, many male health risks are largely preventable and, with changes in attitude, behaviour and lifestyle, men can dramatically reduce their risks. Think of your body as being like a car and treat it with the same care.

Service Your Body Like You Service Your Car

Your Car	Your Body
Tyre pressure	Blood pressure
Oil quality	Blood tests
Water level	Hydration
Fuel consumption	Food and nutrition
Coolant system	Stress levels
Dashboard	Early warning signs of health problems
Braking system	Sleep quality
Locking system	Relaxation
Lights	Eyesight
Indicators	Communication
Spare tyre	Belly fat
Horsepower	Libido
Exhaust pipe	Bowels
Gear stick	Penis
Metallic paint	Skin
Miles on the clock	Exercise
Sat nav	Brain
Steering wheel	Balance centre

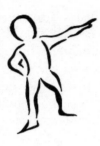

Key Points

- Being an Irish male is a health hazard.
- Irish men die on average about six years earlier than Irish women.
- Many of the serious health conditions affecting men are preventable.
- Have the same respect for your body and mind as you have for your car.
- Remember: prevention is better than cure.
- Your health is your wealth. Treasure it!

2

A Man's Got to Chew
What a Man's Got to Chew

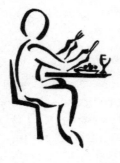 'You are what you eat' is a well-known saying when it comes to eating habits. Most men I know want to eat healthily but they do not want this to be at the cost of enjoying their food. The media is awash with stories about low-fat diets, rapid weight-loss diets, high-carbohydrate diets, low-carbohydrate diets and GI diets (see page 15). The potential information available to us about healthy eating has never been better.

However, at the same time, the consequences of poor eating habits, in the form of obesity and diabetes, are all around us. In the Western world we are in the middle of an epidemic of diabetes and other obesity-related conditions. The basis for preventing these conditions is to have good eating habits. To do that we need to know and understand a little bit about the different food types so that we can make informed food choices for better health. In general terms, a diet rich in natural foods, including lots of fresh fruit and vegetables, whole-grains and fibre, with an emphasis on fish (particularly oily fish), and minimising your intake of animal fat, including red meats, is known to be beneficial. But what about the specifics?

What Is Food?

Food is the source of everything we need to build, maintain and repair our bodies throughout life. Food can provide all the energy, building blocks and nutrition that our bodies need for good health maintenance. Cells in our bodies are continuously repairing and replacing themselves. For example, blood is renewed naturally every ninety days. We need food to give us energy. Everything we do, even sleeping, requires energy, and the source of all our energy is food. Food consists of seven different types of nutrients that our bodies need to function optimally. These are carbohydrates, protein, fat, fibre, water, vitamins and minerals.

Carbohydrates

Carbohydrates provide the main fuel that the body uses for energy. This is called glucose (blood sugar). Carbohydrates are broken down in the stomach into glucose, which then enters the bloodstream. This causes the hormone insulin to be released from the pancreas gland, which enables glucose to be brought into the cells of the body, such as the cells in the muscles, where the sugar can then be used as energy. Carbohydrates are mainly found in fruit and vegetables, pulses and grains. There are two types of carbohydrates: simple carbohydrates and complex carbohydrates.

Simple Carbohydrates

Simple carbohydrates break down quickly after being eaten and enter the bloodstream fast, causing the blood sugar level to rise. Examples of simple carbohydrates include white bread, biscuits and cakes, pure sugar, croissants and fizzy drinks.

Men who eat large amounts of simple carbohydrates can suffer when their blood sugar level goes up and down all day long: the yo-yo effect. Sugar-rich drinks or food causes the blood sugar level to rise very quickly, leading to large amounts of insulin being produced in order to lower the blood sugar and bring some of it into the cells to be used. The excess sugar is turned into fat and can also harm your cholesterol levels. The sudden release of insulin then causes the blood sugar level to drop very quickly. The result is that, an hour or two after eating, your blood sugar level can drop down low, causing feelings of tiredness or weakness and cravings for more sugar-rich carbohydrates, which can start the cycle all over again. The simple way to avoid this and all the problems associated with too many sugar-rich carbohydrates is to eat fewer of them.

Complex Carbohydrates

Complex carbohydrates are much better for us because they are broken down more slowly, thereby causing the blood sugar level to rise more slowly. They tend to keep our blood glucose at a constant level, which helps to optimise our energy levels, decreasing the tendency for carbohydrate cravings and food pangs, and reducing the level of fat deposition. Complex carbohydrates also tend to be quite filling, so they have an added advantage of decreasing any tendency to over-eat. Examples of complex carbohydrates include wholegrain breads and pasta, brown rice and high-fibre cereals such as All-Bran.

The Glycaemic Index (GI)

The glycaemic index is a method of measuring how quickly foods are broken down into sugar. It is easy to understand: glucose itself is given a score of 100 and all other carbohydrates are scored from 1 to 100. Therefore foods with the lowest glycaemic index are complex carbohydrates, which are broken down more slowly, i.e. they don't raise the blood sugar level quickly. By contrast, simple carbohydrates raise the blood sugar quickly and therefore have a high glycaemic index. Research suggests that diets with the highest glycaemic index are associated with an increased risk of diabetes and also lower HDL (good) cholesterol levels (see Chapter 6 for more details on cholesterol). For better health we should concentrate on eating foods with a low GI index. This means the best types of carbohydrates to eat would be oatmeal, wholegrain breads, bran, beans (including kidney beans, soybeans, baked beans and chickpeas), wholegrain pastas and fruit, particularly berries.

Protein

Protein is the body's main building material and is found in foods like meat, eggs, fish, pulses, beans and soy. After eating protein the body breaks down large protein molecules into tiny amino acids and then builds them up again into the protein in the body that is found in hair, teeth, bones, muscles and so on.

A balanced diet will generally give you all the protein you need. You need protein in the body to make your muscles, repair any damage in the body and generally keep the whole system ticking over. Protein is especially important during periods of growth. It helps give power to our muscles and strength to our bones, helps our immune system fight infection, and helps to build us up and keep us strong. Dietary deficiency of protein can cause muscle wasting but this is extremely rare in the Western world, as we only need small amounts of protein in our diets to fulfil our bodies' requirements. In fact, the average 70-kilogram man needs less than 60 grams of protein daily.

Protein is made up of twenty building blocks, known as amino acids. Eleven of these are made in the body, but we need to get the other nine from our diet. If you eat a wide variety of vegetable sources of protein, including beans, rice and various vegetables, then it is possible to get enough of these amino acids. However, if you do not eat a wide enough variety you may become deficient in some of these amino acids. Animal sources of protein, on the other hand, contain all of the amino acids necessary for health. However, the problem with animal sources of protein is that they often contain a lot of fat and cholesterol. Too much animal protein in our diets, i.e. too many burgers and steaks, means too much saturated fat, too much cholesterol and not enough calories from complex carbohydrates and fibre. This can increase your risk for many conditions, including heart disease, colon cancer and diabetes. You should eat protein in moderation and choose low-fat protein sources. Your protein intake should be no more than 10 to 25 per cent of your calorie intake.

The best sources of protein are fish, pulses, egg whites and skinless poultry. It is recommended that you reduce your red meat intake to once or twice a week. Avoid fatty meat or processed meat. So, if you like a good steak, go for the leaner and better cuts, and remember to enjoy it as well. Skim or low-fat milk is a better choice than whole milk. Legumes such as peas, beans and lentils are also good sources of protein and contain less fat than meat and no cholesterol. Soy protein is another useful meat substitute that has many health benefits.

What Is Fat?

Fat is burned as energy and forms a store for future energy needs. It is an important source of fuel: it contains 9 calories per gram, whereas both protein and carbohydrates only contain 4 calories per gram. It is stored in fat reservoirs as a form of fuel. This was ideal in times of famine, but in the Western world today excess fat stores result in unhealthy weight gain and obesity. Fat also helps to insulate the body against heat loss and helps to protect vital organs such as the kidneys. However, the reality is that many of us have too much fat in our diet and consequently store too much of it.

We all need some fat for our bodies to function normally, for our immune systems and hormones, but the problem is that many Irish men eat too much fat, which is quickly converted into blubber and a spare tyre. As well as eating too much fat, many of us eat the wrong type of fat. A high-saturated-fat diet, especially trans-fats (see page 19), creates a build-up of cholesterol and fatty plaques in the blood vessels, which cause narrowing and eventual blockages of the blood vessels, leading to heart attacks and stroke (see Chapters 5 and 6). Reducing your saturated and trans-fat intake is the most important dietary measure you can take to reduce your risk of heart disease. There are several different types of fat, which I call the good, the bad and the ugly.

The Good Fats

Polyunsaturated Fats

These are known as 'essential fatty acids' because they are essential for normal growth and development. The body cannot make either of these essential fatty acids, omega-3 or omega-6.

Omega-3 helps with learning, memory and heart function. Dietary sources of omega-3 include oily fish such as sardines, mackerel, herring and salmon. A healthy diet should contain four times more omega-3 than omega-6.

Omega-6 helps growth, reproduction, coagulation of the blood, healthy skin and the immune system. Good sources of omega-6 include vegetable oils such as sunflower, corn and soy oils, as well as spreads made from these oils, and also meat, nuts and seeds.

Monounsaturated Fats

These are also known as omega-9 and are found in meat, nuts, seeds and olive oil. Dietary sources include meat and meat products, cereals, potato snacks and non-dairy spreads. They are thought to benefit health by suppressing LDL (bad) cholesterol and promoting HDL (good) cholesterol. They are liquid at room temperature.

The Bad Fats

Saturated Fats

These fats increase the risk of heart attack and are know as 'artery cloggers' because they are easily converted by the liver into LDL cholesterol. They are also implicated in many cancers, including colon and prostate cancer. Several vegetable oils, including palm oil, coconut oil and palm kernel oil, are also high in saturated fats and should be avoided. The main dietary sources are full-fat dairy foods, meat and meat products, pastries, biscuits and cakes. Other examples include butter, lard and dripping. Saturated fats are solid at room temperature.

The Ugly Fats

Trans-Fats

Trans-fats, which are also known as hydrogenated fats, have traditionally been found in margarine, vegetable shortening and fried foods. Trans-fats are now banned from many foods and their inclusion in a food must be clearly marked. They are reputedly even worse than saturated fats in terms of promoting heart disease. The World Health Organization warns that no more than 1 per cent of daily energy intake should come from trans-fats. A useful rule of thumb is that 5 grams a day of a trans-fat can raise the risk of heart attack by 25 per cent. You can get more than twice that amount, and in the worst cases more than four times, in a single visit to a fast-food outlet. If you think a diet high in saturated fat is bad for you, and believe me it is, then trans-fats are absolutely deadly. The best way to avoid trans-fats is to read the food labels – avoid hydrogenated fats, trans-fats and partially hydrogenated fats. Even foods labelled 'reduced fat' may contain trans-fats. The best way to reduce satura- ted fats and trans-fats when cooking is to minimise the amount of solid fats you add to food.

See the table below for a guide to fats.

Fat-Based Foods to Choose and Avoid

Choose	Avoid
Olive oil, especially extra virgin olive oil	Grease, lard and gravy
	Trans-fats
Canola oil	Cream sauces
Margarines labelled 'trans-fat free'	Hydrogenated margarine
Cholesterol-lowering spreads	Butter and cocoa butter
	Coconut, palm and cottonseed oils

Fibre

Fibre is an essential part of a healthy diet. It does not have exact nutritional value as it cannot be digested. It is the roughage in veg- etables, grains, fruit and pulses. Fibre helps clear out the bowel, thereby keeping you regular, and also gives you a feeling of fullness, which is an essential part of weight control.

There are two types of fibre. Firstly, there is insoluble fibre, which provides the roughage in our diet, bulking up our stools and helping to keep our bowel motions regular. This prevents constipation and also helps to prevent piles and other conditions of the digestive tract, such as diverticular disease.

Secondly, there is soluble fibre, which is also good at helping to decrease LDL cholesterol levels, while at the same time making us feel full more quickly and slowing the emptying of our stomachs, thus helping to prevent overeating.

Whilst most fibre-rich foods are rich in both insoluble and soluble fibre, there are some food stuffs that are particularly high in soluble fibre. These would include oatmeal (porridge made from oats), fruit such as apricots, prunes, oranges and apples, broccoli, barley, oats, lentils and various types of beans, including soybeans, black beans and kidney beans. While fibre is good for your gut and digestive tract, a diet rich in fibre also helps to decrease the risk of heart disease.

Roughage – The Great Fibre Provider

It is recommended that we eat 30 grams of fibre each day. You can get this by eating a wide variety of wholegrains, fruit and vegetables. Some common fibre-rich foods and their fibre content are listed below.

Fibre-Rich Foods

Type of Food	Fibre Content in Grams (Approximate)
Baked beans (½ cup cooked)	9 grams
Peas (½ cup cooked)	5 grams
1 medium carrot	4 grams
1 medium baked potato (with skin)	4 grams
Oats (1 cup cooked)	3 grams

(Continued)

(Continued)

Type of Food	Fibre Content in Grams (Approximate)
Wholemeal bread (1 slice)	2.46 grams
1 medium tomato	2 grams
Cereals	
All Bran (1 oz)	10 grams
Bran Buds (1 oz)	10 grams
Bran Flakes (1 oz)	5 grams
Corn Flakes (1 oz)	Trace
Dried fruit	
8 figs	19 grams
8 prunes	8 grams
8 apricots	4 grams
Fruit	
1 pear	4 grams
1 apple with skin	4 grams
1 orange	3 grams
1 banana	3 grams

Keys to Getting Enough Fibre

- Start the day well with a high-fibre cereal for breakfast each morning, such as All-Bran, Bran Flakes, Weetabix, muesli or porridge.
- Eat wholemeal bread.
- Eat plenty of fruit and vegetables.
- Eat beans and peas often.
- Stewed fruit is a good source of fibre and is a healthy dessert option.

High-fibre snacks:

- Baked beans on wholemeal toast
- Vegetable or lentil soup and wholemeal bread
- Mixed dried fruit and nuts
- Wholemeal scone and jam
- Stewed prunes and custard
- High-fibre breakfast cereals and milk

Water

Water is an essential part of all the processes that go on throughout the body. Our bodies need plenty of water to keep every system ticking over. We need to drink plenty of fluids on a daily basis to stay healthy and the best fluid of all is water. Generally it is recommended to drink about six to eight glasses per day. The key is to stay well hydrated. The best guide to hydration status is the colour of your urine, which should be clear. Thirst, on the other hand, is a poor indicator of hydration – you can be a litre or more behind in your fluids before thirst starts to kick in.

Tea – Are You Having a Cuppa?

Drinking tea appears to be good for your health. This is because tea contains substances called polyphenols, which are powerful antioxidants that help to keep cells in the body healthy and protect against the ravaging effects of oxygen-free radicals, which are associated with cancer and heart disease. Tea also contains caffeine. However, the caffeine in tea appears to be absorbed into your system much more slowly than caffeine from coffee, which means that brain activity is stimulated for a much longer time. Tea contains a number of vitamins and minerals. There is some evidence that drinking black tea reduces your risk of heart disease and has a generally positive effect on health. Green tea appears to be even better for you as it contains more of the protective polyphenols than black tea. Green tea is thought to have many health benefits, including helping to prevent heart disease and cancer. Because green tea is drunk without milk or sugar and is naturally free of calories and salt, it is an excellent choice as part of a calorie-controlled diet. It is also excellent for relieving stress.

The jury is out on coffee in terms of health effects. Certainly, in moderation coffee is unlikely to be harmful. However, the caffeine in coffee is a stimulant and, while many of us may need a cup or two to get going in the morning, excess caffeine can cause your system to speed up, sometimes aggravating stress symptoms or causing palpitations. Just like alcohol, the story with coffee may be another case of 'less is more'.

What About Vitamins?

Vitamins are small molecules that play a key role in your overall physical and mental well-being. There are two types of vitamins. Firstly, there are the water-soluble vitamins, which are not stored in the body and are flushed out in the urine each day. Therefore, it is important to get enough of the water-soluble vitamins on a daily basis to prevent possible deficiency occurring. These include Vitamin C and eight different types of B vitamins. Secondly, there are the fat-soluble vitamins, which include Vitamins A, D, E and K. These vitamins can be stored in fat cells in the body for future use so it is not essential to get the exact amount each and every day to prevent deficiency occurring.

We know 'an apple a day keeps the doctor away'. Should we all be taking a multivitamin? I believe the answer is yes for most Irish men. There is no doubt that a diet full of fresh fruit and vegetables, and high in fibre, wholegrains and oily fish, will give people most of the vitamins they require. However, many Irish men, for one reason or another, do not get their recommended intake of fruit and vegetables. Therefore I think a good general multivitamin can be invaluable. The following vitamins are particularly relevant in the context of men's health:

- Folic acid (Vitamin B$_9$) – this has been known for many years to be of benefit to women of child-bearing age to prevent spina bifida in their children. However, in recent years folic acid has been shown to help prevent heart attacks, by lowering the level of a chemical called homocysteine in the blood stream, which can cause hardening of the arteries. Folic acid may also have a role in helping to prevent cancer.
- Vitamins B$_6$ and B$_{12}$ – these also help lower levels of homocysteine and therefore may help decrease the risk of heart attack.
- Vitamin D – this vitamin is essential to keep the bones strong by allowing calcium to be absorbed from the gut and into the bones. Foods rich in Vitamin D include oily fish, milk with added Vitamin D, margarine, eggs and liver. Our skin can make our own Vitamin D if we get enough sunlight. But as we get older the skin is less able to produce it, so older people need to eat foods rich in Vitamin D or take a Vitamin D supplement. However, it is not easy to get enough Vitamin D from dietary sources alone so it is useful to include it in your multivitamin supplement.
- Niacin (Vitamin B$_3$) – this can also be a very helpful supplement in the battle to lower cholesterol. Niacin works by raising the HDL (good) cholesterol level by up to 30 per cent while at the same time lowering the LDL (bad) cholesterol level. Niacin can also significantly lower blood fat (triglyceride) levels. However, generally speaking, high doses of niacin are needed to produce these effects and niacin in high doses can cause side effects including facial flushing, skin itching, headaches and other more serious side effects. Therefore, if you are considering using high-dose niacin you should first discuss it with your family doctor.

Minerals

Minerals are substances (inorganic ions) that are involved in a whole range of bodily functions and are essential for good health. There are about eighteen different minerals, found widely in food. Only tiny amounts of many of these minerals are needed for good health. Indeed, some are needed in such tiny amounts that it is nearly impossible to be deficient in them if you eat a balanced diet.

A mineral we need a lot of is calcium because it is so important for our bone structure, as our bones have a high calcium content. Dietary sources of calcium include dairy products such as milk, yogurt and cheese, as well as brown bread, broccoli and oily fish like sardines. Most other minerals such as iron, fluoride and manganese are only needed in very tiny quantities. Zinc is a mineral of particular importance for men's reproductive health as it is needed for male fertility and the proper manufacture of sperm. It also helps the immune system and with promoting the healing of wounds. Zinc is found in seafood, turkey, wholegrains, oatmeal, eggs, yeast, nuts and beans.

The Food Pyramid

The food pyramid gives a good idea of how our daily food intake should be balanced. Understanding the food pyramid can help you keep your diet varied and interesting, while at the same time remaining healthy.

1. The bottom row is the *carbohydrate group*, with food that supplies us with energy in the form of glucose. This includes cereal, bread, potatoes, pasta, rice and grains. This is the largest group and six or more portions are recommended each day (up to twelve portions if you are very active). Wholegrains should be chosen where possible.

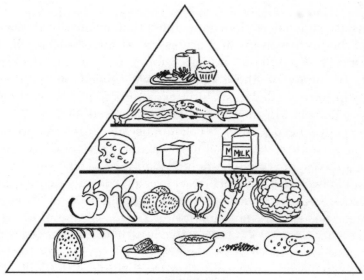

FOOD PYRAMID

Wholegrains

These foods are a good source of fibre and complex carbohydrates. Wholegrains are also a good source of vitamins and minerals, which are beneficial for maintaining a healthy blood pressure level and heart health. These include selenium, zinc, magnesium, iron, niacin, riboflavin, thiamine and Vitamin E.

As an example, brown rice has the same fat, protein and calories as white rice but also has additional fibre, calcium, iron, zinc and folic acid as well as Vitamins B_1, B_2 and B_6. It can help normalise blood sugar and is thought to be particularly good for the bowel, perhaps helping to lower the risk of bowel cancer. It can also lower blood cholesterol levels.

Ground flaxseed is an excellent way to add wholegrain to your diet. These small brown seeds can be crushed or ground in a food processor or coffee maker and added to food, e.g. a teaspoonful in hot cereal or yogurt. Flax seeds are high in fibre and also in omega-3.

Simple ways to increase the amount of wholegrains in your diet are shown below.

How to Increase Your Wholegrain Intake

Choose	Avoid
Brown rice	White rice
High-fibre cereals	Sugar-loaded cereals
Oats	Muffins and doughnuts
Whole wheat pasta	Regular pasta
100 per cent wholegrain breads	Bread made with white flour
Bake with whole wheat flour	White flour
Add ground flaxseed to your diet	

2. *Fruit and vegetables* make up the second largest group in the food pyramid and it is recommended that we eat at least five portions of fruit and vegetables per day. We should all eat more fresh fruit and vegetables. However, many Irish men fall short on this one. Fruit and vegetables are excellent for your health for a number of reasons. Firstly, they are an excellent source of vitamins and minerals and are naturally low in calories. Secondly, they are high in soluble fibre, which can lower cholesterol and help prevent heart disease. Thirdly, fresh fruit and vegetables are very rich in antioxidants, which can help prevent heart disease and cancer. Berries are a particularly rich natural source of antioxidants, especially blueberries. Broccoli is a rich vegetable source of antioxidants and as such is called a 'superfood' (see page 29). Fourthly, they can be quite filling, which means less space for high-fat foods.

The key with fruit and vegetables is to eat them often, ideally with every meal. Keeping fresh fruit in a bowl in the kitchen or freshly chopped carrots or broccoli in the fridge makes a healthy snack readily available. The only fruit and vegetables to avoid would be vegetables in creamy sauces, fried vegetables in batter and canned fruit with heavy sweet syrup. Otherwise, for fruit and veg the sky's the limit.

What Are Superfoods?

These are foods such as fruit and vegetables that are very high in antioxidants. Examples include berries, especially blueberries, and broccoli. The high level of antioxidants in these foods helps protect the body against the damage that oxygen-free radicals can do to our bodies. This can help reduce the risk of many conditions, including cancers and heart disease, and can potentially slow down the very ageing process itself.

Oxygen-free radicals are produced in the body when we burn energy. They are also very prevalent in certain foods, for example, processed food and fried foods. These oxygen-free radicals are thought to damage the body in various ways. They can cause LDL cholesterol to become stickier and lead to hardening of the lining of the blood vessel walls, causing narrowing and eventually potential blockages of these arteries. They can affect the integrity of the immune system, with oxygen-free radicals allowing the unregulated growth of cancer cells.

Antioxidants are the subject of considerable ongoing research to see what role they may play in health, wellness and disease prevention. Keep yourself informed about developments in this area in the years ahead.

3. The *dairy group* of foods is next in the food pyramid and two or three portions a day is recommended to give us enough calcium and Vitamin D for strong bones and teeth.
4. The *protein group* is next and again two or three portions daily are recommended to provide enough protein and iron. The best

sources are oily fish or chicken rather than red meat. Eggs, beans, pulses and soy are also part of this group.

Soy is a vegetable protein that is eaten widely in the Far East. Soy seems to have many health benefits. It is rich in the B vitamins, potassium, calcium, fibre, protein and also some of the good fats that are actually good for your heart. Soy also has substances called isoflavones, which may be good for the prostate in terms of helping to prevent prostate cancer.

5. The smallest group is at the top. This is the area reserved for sweets, treats, high-fat snack foods and other *junk food*. A little every so often is okay but portions should be small relative to the other food groupings.

What is in ONE Portion?

Grains

- one bowl of breakfast cereal
- one slice of bread
- two tablespoons of cooked pasta/rice
- one medium potato – boiled or baked

Fruit and Vegetables

- two tablespoons of cooked vegetables or salad
- a small bowl of homemade vegetable soup
- one medium-sized piece of fresh fruit
- a small bowl of chopped or canned fruit
- a glass of fruit/vegetable juice (6 oz)

Dairy

- one cup of milk
- one yoghurt

- 1 oz of cheese

Protein

- 2 to 3 oz of meat, chicken or fish
- two eggs (ideally not more than seven per week)
- six tablespoons of cooked peas/beans
- 2 oz of cheddar-type cheese
- 3 oz of nuts

The Good Guys – Foods to Live For

- Eat lots of fresh fruit and vegetables for vitamins, minerals and fibre. Eat more potassium-rich foods such as bananas, citrus fruits and other fruit and vegetables. Complex carbohydrates, found in wholegrains, vegetables and fruit, are your best energy source.
- Eat foods with a low glycaemic index (GI).
- Make sure you get your recommended daily allowances for your vitamins and minerals.
- Eat more calcium-rich foods such as broccoli, spinach, tofu and low-fat dairy products.
- Eat probiotic yoghurts. These can boost the immune system, prevent yeast infections, and raise good cholesterol and lower bad cholesterol. They are also rich in calcium, which is good for your bones, can help prevent bad breath and may have some benefits for the digestive tract.
- Eat more fibre. Eat at least 30 grams of fibre per day, especially sources of soluble fibre such as oats, barley and beans. Eat more pulses, such as lentils, black-eyed beans, cannelloni beans and chickpeas. These are low in fat and high in fibre, vitamins, protein and minerals.

- Switch to fish instead of red meat. Eat more fish, especially cold-water oily fish such as salmon, tuna, sardines and mackerel. These are all rich sources of omega-3, a fish oil that is very good for your heart. Fish is a good source of protein and doesn't have the saturated fat that red meat contains.
- Drink six to eight glasses of water a day and keep your urine clear in colour.
- Limit your alcohol consumption to no more than 21 units per week.
- If you like a little indulgence then consider dark chocolate. Chocolate with a cocoa content of 70 per cent or higher is full of flavinoids and other powerful antioxidants. As a treat, a square or two is not a bad option.

The Bad Guys – Foods to Avoid

- Eat less fat. Reducing your dietary intake of both saturated fat and trans-fat is the most important dietary measure you can take to reduce your risk of heart disease.
- Avoid processed foods where possible.
- Eat less sugary foods and avoid refined sugar where possible.
- Avoid 'stodgy carbs' such as white bread, cakes, pies, doughnuts, crisps, buttered popcorn, biscuits and muffins.
- Eat protein in moderation and choose low-fat protein sources.
- Reduce your sodium salt intake to less than one teaspoon (2400 milligrams) per day.

Salt

Excess dietary salt can help cause high blood pressure, which is an important risk factor for heart disease and stroke. We can become tolerant to the taste of salt and unwittingly use more and more over time to get the same taste (just like with sugar).

Steps to reduce salt intake include avoiding table salt. Be aware of high sources of salt such as tinned soups, soy sauce and frozen dinners. Remember that processed foods tend to be very high in salt; these include snack foods, frozen meals, tinned foods and cheese. Instead of using salt in cooking, consider other herbs and flavoursome spices. Watch the salt content of sauces and consider salt substitutes, for example, sea salt, but use sparingly.

Breakfast Like a King

Breakfast is the most important meal of the day. Yet many men don't eat any breakfast because they are 'too busy'. Research has shown that those who eat a good breakfast tend to perform better, both physically and mentally, than those who choose to skip the meal. It makes sense, as getting a nutritious, healthy breakfast will give you lots of energy and keep your brain alert and active. Forget the breakfast rolls or the artery-clogging full Irish. Instead go for a bowl of fibre-rich cereal and skim milk or some fruit. The protein in the milk will help to invigorate your brain, while the complex carbohydrates in the cereal and fruit will give you long-lasting energy until lunchtime.

How To Improve Your Diet and Nutrition

- It is important to focus on eating plenty of foods that are good for you. This is a positive lifestyle choice that can have huge knock-on benefits for your health.
- Knowledge precedes awareness and awareness precedes change. The first step is to know what your nutritional needs are. Having read this chapter you should have better knowledge of the types of foods you need to eat to keep your body healthy.
- Keep a food diary of everything you eat and drink, not just what but also when, where and why. Keep the diary for a week or so

and include a weekend. Many's the healthy eating habit that goes by the wayside come Friday evening. Be honest with yourself and try to answer the following questions: Do you comfort eat? Do you tend to shop when you are hungry? Do you eat a good breakfast? Do you eat 'on the run'? Keeping a food diary should give you invaluable insight into your current dietary habits and highlight the areas that need change.

- Decide on what changes you are going to make. Try to keep these changes positive ones, such as 'I am going to eat a better breakfast,' 'I am going to eat more fish' or 'I am going to eat less animal fat.'
- Try to focus on some specific realistic targets that you can set for yourself. By focusing on eating foods that are good for you, you leave less time and space for eating bad stuff. Keeping a dietary record allows you to monitor your progress. It is important to reward yourself regularly for the success achieved.
- Finally, be realistic. No one is perfect. We all have the occasional blowout and that in itself is no bad thing. As the saying goes, moderation in all things, including moderation. Stay on track with your healthy lifestyle as it is what you do 90 per cent of the time that counts in the long run.

We all have our excuses: too busy, too little time, etc. But if we truly value our health, then we must give our bodies the best fuel possible to keep the engine ticking over. Don't use excuses for not following a healthy eating plan. Your health is too important for that.

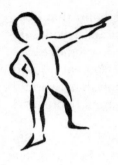

Key Points

- There are seven different types of nutrients found in food; we need to consume all of these nutrients in the correct amounts to keep our bodies energised and healthy.
- Plan ahead.
- Breakfast like a king.
- Eat a wide variety of foods.
- Emphasise wholegrains as well as fresh fruit and vegetables.
- Choose lean protein sources.
- Limit high-fat and salty foods.
- Improving your diet is a great start to a healthier you.

3

When Size Really Does Matter

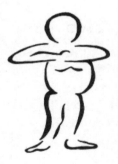 Obesity and weight-related health problems are the new epidemics in twenty-first century Ireland. Obesity is now almost as bad as cigarette smoking as a major preventable cause of premature death.

Obesity is defined as excess body fat. In men, body fat tends to accumulate particularly around the belly area and upper chest, which increases the chances of heart attack and stroke. In addition, the explosion of diabetes in recent years is directly related to the increase in the number of people suffering from obesity.

The amount of body fat you have and where it is distributed is very important for your health. What you weigh is less important than where that weight is distributed.

Some Scary Facts and Figures

- Over 60 per cent of Irish men are either overweight or obese.
- About two-fifths of Irish men are overweight and one-quarter of Irish men are obese.

- The trend towards obesity is increasing and it is estimated that by the year 2050 up to 60 per cent of Irish men may be obese.

Apples and Pears

Did you know that the shape of your body can be directly related to your later risk of ill-health? Pear-shaped people tend to store fat around their hips and thighs while apple-shaped people store fat around their bellies. This apple shape, known as central obesity, increases your risk of heart disease, diabetes and ill health. Big bellies beware!

What Are the Health Consequences of Being Overweight or Obese?

Obesity is associated with a whole range of physical conditions, including heart disease, high blood pressure, diabetes, arthritis, gall stones, hernia, varicose veins and several cancers, including bowel cancer. In addition, obesity may be associated with a range of psychological issues, including low self-esteem, poor body image and depression.

What Causes Obesity?

In the vast majority of cases, being overweight or obese is due to a simple mismatch between the amount of energy consumed, in the form of food and beverages, and the amount of energy expended, in the form of exercise. A typical adult male requires 2,000–2,500 calories a day, depending on age. The calorie requirements get lower as we get older. It is believed that 1 pound of fat equates to about 3,000 excess calories.

For many men the increased demands of work, career and family life mean that exercise habits and sporting interests often keenly pursued during the teens and early twenties get put to one side. The result is that much less energy is burned up. The sedentary lifestyle of modern living can mean hours in the car and sitting watching television with no opportunity to burn calories. Combine this with a high-fat diet of large portions and lots of processed food and the effects can be lethal. Even subtle lifestyle changes over time can lead to a net gain in terms of calories consumed. These excess calories are stored in the body as fat. A small increase in calorie intake (food or drink) combined with a small reduction in activity or exercise levels leads to net weight gain over time.

People often talk about weight problems being due to their metabolism but really it is about being active enough to burn up the calories or energy you take in each day in the form of food and drink. The best way to improve your metabolism is to exercise because regular exercise will allow you to burn up energy and fat more quickly.

Is It My Genes, Doctor?

Obesity can run in families. Fat parents often have fat children and the reasons for this may be due to family dietary and exercise habits and attitudes to food, as well as lifestyle and behaviour. However, the possibility of a 'fat gene' is the subject of much research. This fat gene may have given people a survival advantage in famine times. Nowadays, though, having a fat gene may mean you can't break down fat and sugars properly and you have a tendency to store fat. This definitely increases your likelihood of becoming obese. So if weight problems run in your family, beware. Forewarned is forearmed.

Obesity is also linked with educational status and socioeconomic group. In the nineteenth century, fatness was a sign of wealth and status, whereas in the twenty-first century Western world it is now associated with poverty.

The sedentary lifestyle and high-fat, large-portion diets of the Western world, so-called modern living, is helping to ensure that each generation is heavier than the last. This is called 'passive obesity'.

Psychological and emotional factors govern our thoughts and feelings towards food. Comfort eating or a tendency to binge eat can also be factors in obesity. Much rarer causes of obesity would include medical conditions that affect the metabolism, such as an underactive thyroid gland or Cushing's syndrome.

Key Measurements

Waist Circumference

Size does matter and measuring your abdominal circumference or girth with a tape measure is a reliable indicator of whether you are overweight or not. This is perhaps the most accurate indicator of central obesity, in other words the amount of fat stored around the belly. The bottom line is that excess fat around your waist means a greater risk of future health problems. This can be measured using a simple tape measure. Wrap it around from your back to your front at the level of the belly button. As a man, your waist circumference should be less than 37 inches. A waist circumference greater than 40 inches is definitely bad news and increases your risk of many health conditions, including heart disease. The higher your waist goes over 40 inches the greater the risk.

Measuring your waist accurately:

- Place a tape measure around your belly above the level of the hip bones at the belly button.
- Make sure it is level all the way around
- Relax and measure your waist after you breathe out.
- No sucking in your belly and make sure the tape measure is snug but not so tight that it pushes into the skin.

Remember that your waist measurement is not the same as the size trousers you wear. Some men are astounded when their waists are measured and discover, for example, it's 42 inches and protest, 'Sure I only wear a 38 inch waist!'

Body Mass Index (BMI)

This measurement has been used since the nineteenth century to predict the likelihood of health risks from excess weight. It is calculated by dividing your weight in kilos by your height in metres, squared. For example a man who is 5'10" in height and weighs 13 stone and 7 pounds has a BMI of 27, which is calculated as follows:

Weight (13st 7lb) = 86kg; Height (5'10") = 1.78 metres
$$BMI = 86/(1.78)^2 = 27$$

Significance of BMI

BMI	Classed As	Health Risk
Less than 18.5	Underweight	Some health risk
18.5 to 24.9	Ideal	Normal
25 to 29.9	Overweight	Moderate health risk
30 to 39.9	Obese	High health risk
40 and over	Very obese	Very high health risk

BMI is used widely by insurance companies for actuarial purposes, in the context of life insurance, etc. While it is not an exact science, your BMI does give a fairly reliable indication of potential health risks associated with your weight. It has recently come in for some criticism as it is less accurate in athletic muscular men and the elderly.

Athletic men who are quite muscular can have a lot of heavy muscle but very little body fat. Their BMI tends to be falsely elevated. So they can have a higher BMI category even though their level of body fat is normal.

On the other hand, elderly people tend to have less muscle so their BMI can be misleading. In other words, a normal BMI in an elderly man doesn't rule out obesity-related problems. Waist-to-hip ratio and belly size are much more significant in this age group.

Middle-Age Spread

In early middle age, an expanding waistline is accompanied by a rise in weight. However, as men get older and muscle turns into fat (which is lighter than muscle), you may be making and depositing more fat and yet the scales may remain the same. Therefore don't rely too much on your weight alone or your BMI as you get older. Watch your waistline, which is a better guide to your fat stores and risk of health-related problems.

Waist-to-Hip Ratio

Your waist-to-hip ratio is a figure calculated by dividing your waist size by your hip size in inches. The upper acceptable limit for men is 0.9. There is a significantly increased risk of heart attack and stroke in men with a waist-to-hip ratio greater than 1. This measurement is more relevant than BMI in men over 75 years of age.

Know Your Numbers

The two key numbers to know with regard to your size are your BMI, which should be less than 25, and your abdominal circumference, which should be less than 37 inches. If they are below these thresholds, chances are you are in reasonable shape. If not, then it is never too late to make some positive changes to get your weight down. Remember, losing a little can make a big difference.

How to Measure Body Fat

Measurement of body fat can by done by using a body fat callipers and taking measurements of three areas of your body: your biceps area on the front of your arm, your triceps area at the back of your arm, and your abdominal or tummy area. By doing this you can calculate your percentage body fat using an age-adjusted table. Alternatively there are scanners available that can give a detailed and accurate analysis of body fat.

The Obesity Time Bomb – Why a Big Belly is Bad for Your Health

A big belly – excess body fat stored around the belly area – increases the risk of ill-health. Quite simply you increase your risk of developing some or all of the following medical conditions. These risks are increased significantly if your waist circumference is over 40 inches. So if you are apple-shaped – watch out.

- Heart disease, including heart attack and angina
- Stroke
- Higher cholesterol levels
- Gall stones
- Some cancers, particularly bowel cancer and prostate cancer
- Osteoarthritis, especially of the weight-bearing joints such as the hips and knees. One pound of fat around the belly puts *ten* pounds of pressure on the hips and knees. So, if you are carrying 10 pounds of excess fat around your belly, this will put pressure of 100 pounds on your weight-bearing joints.
- High blood pressure. Every extra pound of fat you have needs a blood supply. If you were to get all the tiny thread-like blood vessels supplying that pound of fat and stretch them out into an imaginary line, you would have an extra mile. So if you are 3

stone overweight this means your heart has to pump blood an extra 42 miles every time it beats. You can see how this can cause your blood pressure to go up over time.

- Sleep apnoea syndrome. This is where snorers develop pauses or absences in their breathing due to effects on the breathing centre in the brain. Obesity is a big risk factor.
- Gastro–oesophageal reflux disease (heartburn). This is where acid comes back up the food pipe from the stomach, causing belching, heartburn or indigestion.
- Higher complication rates from surgery, including wound infection, chest infection and clotting in the legs (deep vein thrombosis). Operations such as hip replacement surgery can be more difficult.
- Diabetes. In simple terms the pancreas gland, which is the organ responsible for regulating blood sugar levels through the pro- duction of insulin, becomes burnt out through shear overwork. Symptoms of diabetes include fatigue, thirst and urinating more frequently. In middle-aged men diabetes can be present for several years before a diagnosis is made. So if you are overweight and have any of these symptoms consult your family doctor.
- Metabolic syndrome – this is where a person has a group of risk factors that significantly increase their risk of diabetes and heart disease. If you have at least three of the following features then you have metabolic syndrome:

  o a waist circumference greater than 40 inches
  o raised blood pressure (greater than 130 over 85)
  o raised fasting blood sugar (an indication of diabetes)
  o raised blood fat (triglycerides) levels
  o low levels of HDL cholesterol (the good or happy cholesterol – see Chapter 6), i.e. HDL levels less than 1

The presence of any three of the above-listed factors diagnoses metabolic syndrome, which means you are at increased risk of developing heart disease, diabetes, stroke or all three.

The Health Benefits of Losing Weight

If an obese man can lose 10 per cent of his body weight there are major health gains (10 per cent of body weight in many cases would be about 10 kilograms, which is about 22 pounds):

- You may need to take less medication.
- Psychological benefits – you may feel better and have a better quality of life.
- You can reduce your chance of dying from obesity-related conditions.
- If you have high blood pressure, you can reduce your pressure by 10 mmHg (see Chapter 5). A blood pressure of 140/90 can become 130/80, which may help avoid the need for long-term medication.
- If your fasting blood sugar level is raised (known as impaired glucose tolerance), then you can reduce your chances significantly of getting diabetes. If you have diabetes your blood sugars will be lower and you will be better able to control your diabetes.
- Your cholesterol levels will improve: your total cholesterol and LDL (bad) cholesterol levels will decrease and your HDL (good) cholesterol levels can increase.

What Should I Do if I am Overweight or Obese?

The key to losing weight and body fat can be summed up in one word: action. Knowledge and understanding always precede change.

Informing yourself about the health issues relating to weight and obesity allows you to make informed choices. Simply measuring your belly circumference with a tape measure will give you a reasonable picture of where you are. Understanding the health risks and also the huge benefits of taking action can be a great stimulus for positive change.

Of course the challenge is to make some positive changes that will improve your overall health. The only reliable way to lose excess weight and body fat is to burn up fat by regular physical exercise (preferably daily) and to reduce your calorie intake by focusing on healthy eating patterns.

Some Keys to Reducing Weight and Body Fat:

- It is not easy to lose body fat and there is no quick fix.
- Keep a food, mood and exercise diary. I think it is useful to keep a detailed diary over the course of a week of everything you eat and drink, including alcohol, and also a record of your exercise levels. Keeping a record of your mood as well will allow you to see if comfort eating can be a factor for you, as some men tend to eat more or drink more alcohol if they are under stress. This can help give you insight into not only what you eat but also the where, when and why. Reflect on how you feel at times when you eat. Do you comfort eat? If so, learn to create a number of new coping strategies, such as drinking a pint of water or going for a walk instead.
- Don't skip meals, especially breakfast. Meals should not be skipped as hunger pangs can then set in, which can greatly lower one's resistance to chocolate and high-fat snacks. 'Breakfast like a king, lunch like a prince and sup like a pauper' – this old saying

is very true. From personal experience I know that many people with weight problems don't eat a decent breakfast and make up for this by piling in lots of excess calories, often late into the night. Breakfast is the most important meal of the day and can give your day a great start.

- Focus on eating foods that are good for you. This leaves less time and space for the bad stuff. Eating complex carbohydrates, wholegrains, lots of fruit and vegetables, and lots of fibre-rich foods helps to keep the blood sugar level constant, which is good for your metabolism. Focus on healthy snacks.
- It is important to decrease your intake of fat. Focus on reducing the fat content of your diet, as a portion of fat contains twice as many calories as the same weighted portion of protein or carbohydrates.
- Limit your portion size.
- Drink plenty of water or low-calorie drinks (avoid high-sugar drinks).
- Reduce your alcohol intake. Alcohol is fattening: it has calories that are empty – in other words of non-nutritional value – and alcohol often lowers the blood sugar levels, which can bring on hunger pangs.
- Stay positive and focus on positive changes that you can maintain. Don't weigh yourself too often as small fluctuations in weight can be due to fluid retention.
- Plan ahead. Keep your cupboards stocked with healthy foods, including healthy snack options. Don't shop when you are hungry.
- Be realistic. Aim for 1 to 2 pounds of weight loss per week. If you lose weight more quickly than this you will tend to lose

muscle as well. Five hundred calories less per day equates to about one stone in weight lost over about three months.

- Consider involving others. Support groups like Weight Watchers can provide terrific support. Traditionally Weight Watchers was only for women, but now men are wakening up to the huge value of group support. There is no need to soldier on alone. Involve your friends in your new healthier lifestyle. Many hands make light work.

- Combine these sensible eating habits with a vigorous exercise programme. Exercise has tremendous health benefits, which include improving your metabolism to help you to burn fat. While 30 minutes per day is needed for good health, to lose weight you should aim for 45 to 60 minutes per day. The best results come from small changes that you can stick to rather than dramatic changes that only last a week or so. Remember, each journey begins with a single step!

Can You Reduce Your Belly Fat with Sit-Ups?

Sit-ups will strengthen your stomach wall muscles, which can help you to tone them. However, they won't reduce your belly fat. The good news is that all exercise, especially aerobic exercise, which gets your heart rate and breathing up, is good to help you burn fat. Many men will lose belly fat before they lose fat elsewhere on the body.

Fad Diets – False Promises

You may have heard or read about it many times. Some new diet promises amazing weight loss in a short period of time with guaranteed results: 'lose 20 pounds in 2 weeks'. Fad diets tend to promise dramatic results in terms of weight loss and altered body shape. This can sound tempting, particularly when these adverts are accompanied by pictures showing 'before' and 'after' photos.

However, if it sounds too good to be true then it probably is. These diets are usually bad for your health and in the long run generally do not work. They are popular because they offer a 'quick fix', relatively pain-free solution. In the short term people often do lose weight on these diets, but this weight loss tends to be caused by the loss of bodily fluids and lean muscle. Food choices are generally limited and, as variety is the spice of life, most people pack in these diets after a few weeks.

The reality is that the vast majority of people regain the weight they have lost over a short period of time. Indeed, most people who lose weight initially on fad diets end up putting on more than they lost. There are two reasons for this. Firstly, crash diets generally deprive us of adequate amounts of food, so, to compensate for this, our metabolism slows down, burning up less and less energy in an attempt to conserve fat stores. This is what happens to bears when they hibernate during the winter months. The problem is that when our metabolism slows down we burn less energy, meaning that smaller amounts of food can cause weight gain. Secondly, good old human nature causes fad diets to fail. For most of us, eating is one of the most pleasurable things in life. No one likes to be deprived of pleasurable eating for too long. Very few people can stick to a diet of boiled vegetables and carrot juice for long, no matter how promising the results.

The key to successful weight loss in the longer term is a combination of sensible eating habits and high activity levels to keep the metabolism up.

How to Cut Down on Fat

Fat can add taste and flavour to many foods. A certain amount of fat is okay, maybe up to 20 per cent of our dietary calorie requirements. However, the problem is most of us eat far more than this.

Tips to cut fat from your diet:

- Avoid fried food. Instead boil, bake, poach or steam food. Cook vegetables in water and herbs instead of butter or oil.
- If you eat canned tuna, eat the type packed in brine rather than oil.
- Use only fat-free or low-fat dairy products.
- If you eat red meat use only lean portions. Better still, eat fish or white meat without the skin.
- For salad dressings try oil-free ones like plain lemon juice mixed with balsamic vinegar.
- Avoid adding butter to your food.
- Avoid pasties and rich desserts such as cheesecake.
- Check the labels on food packets carefully.
- Avoid eating fatty foods at night when your ability to digest and burn up food drops significantly. Also you are not exercising to burn it up.
- Develop and maintain sensible eating habits.
- Try to eat only seated at the table.
- Use a smaller plate and take smaller portions.
- Be organised – bring your own low-fat lunch to work with you, for example, wholemeal sandwiches with lean tuna or chicken, and some fruit.
- Remember, don't get too fanatical – small, simple, steady steps you can maintain are much better than a week or two of misery followed by breaking out.

More information about healthy eating and keeping fit can be found in Chapters 2 and 4.

Sensible Substitutes for High-Fat Foods

High-Fat Food	Sensible Substitute
Ice cream	Frozen fat-free yoghurt or sorbet
Butter	Olive oil
Mayonnaise	Fat-free mayonnaise
Cream-based soups	Broth-based soups
Chocolate chip cookies	Fig rolls and ginger snaps
Doughnuts	Wholemeal scone
Roasted peanuts	Raisins
Whole-milk products, including milk, yoghurt and full-fat cheeses	Skimmed or low-fat milk, yoghurt, cottage cheese and reduced fat cheeses

Snacking

There is some evidence that eating regularly can allow you better control over your weight and help you to be leaner. Eating a healthy snack between meals can be good for your health as well as your waistline. A healthy snack can help to ward off hunger pangs, maintain a constant blood sugar level and keep the engine burning fuel at a steady pace. It can also help to reduce the number of calories you consume at meal times. If you are less hungry you may not feel like diving into the bread or having second helpings. Of course, it is important to watch the portion size of a snack so it doesn't turn into a meal in itself. Examples of sensible snacks include:

- Fresh fruit
- Dried apricots
- Raisins/sultanas
- 1/2 cup of yogurt mixed with 1/2 cup of fresh or frozen berries
- rice cakes
- Low-fat fruit yogurt

51

- A small bowl of breakfast cereal with skimmed milk
- Wholemeal scone – fruit or plain
- Berry smoothie

Drug Treatments for Obesity

Medication has a limited role to play in the management of obesity. These drugs should only be used when a lifestyle programme of dietary change combined with exercise has been tried first, ideally for several months. At this stage a trial of medication may be considered if further weight loss is needed. The use of these drugs should follow strict criteria and guidelines, which include:

- An initial three-month trial with weight-reducing diet and exercise
- Your BMI must be 30 or above, or
- Your BMI must be 28 or above, and you have a definite medical condition that would benefit from you losing weight (such as diabetes or high blood pressure)
- You should lose at least 5 per cent of your weight within three months of starting and at least 10 per cent of your weight after six months. If not, the medication should be stopped.

There are currently two such medications available in Ireland. Orlistat (Xenical) works in two ways. Firstly, it helps to block the absorption of fat from food in your gut so that less fat gets into the body. Secondly, this undigested fat is then passed out with your faeces (stools), which are more slimy, fatty and can be quite offensive and smelly, which can act as a further deterrent to eating fatty foods.

Sibutramine (Reductil) acts on the appetite centre in the brain. It works by reducing your appetite and making you feel full more quickly. The result is that you feel more 'full' with less food. You should not take sibutramine if you have high blood pressure or a heart condition. Careful and regular monitoring of blood pressure and pulse rate is important for anyone taking this medication and it must be discontinued if these start to increase.

Do These Drugs Work?

The current evidence suggests that these drugs, when combined with a healthy lifestyle, can lead to more weight loss than a weight-reducing diet and exercise alone. The effectiveness of these drugs can vary widely from person to person. One reason why these drugs may not work is that you may be tempted to throw in the towel on the healthy lifestyle if you think a pill is going to sort it all out for you. None of these drugs are guaranteed to make you lose weight. You still have to continue to eat a healthy weight-reducing diet, and to exercise as much as possible.

Surgery

This can be an option for men with severe obesity, or moderate obesity and another medical condition such as diabetes or sleep apnoea. There are several types of weight-loss surgery. The most common type is called lap banding, where by a band is placed around the stomach so that you feel full more quickly, resulting in a smaller intake of food. Another type of surgery is known as a gastric bypass, in which a small pouch allows food to bypass the stomach and go straight into the bowel, which means you feel fuller after less food and you also tend to absorb fewer calories. Surgical treatment can help someone to lose a considerable amount of their excess weight. However, these procedures can cause complications and should only be done by a specialist in the area. It is also important to follow a healthy lifestyle programme after surgery.

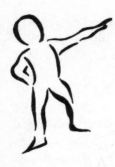

Key Points

- Obesity is a major health issue for Irish men.
- Complications of obesity can include diabetes and heart disease.
- To prevent obesity:
  - maintain high levels of physical activity
  - eat regular meals, especially breakfast
  - be consistent with your eating habits – on weekends as well as weekdays
- Everything in moderation; don't feel guilty if you have the occasional slip. It's what you do 90 per cent of the time that's important.
- Monitor your waist as well as your weight.
- Avoid fad diets.
- Stay positive.

4

Exercise –
Probably the Best Pill of All

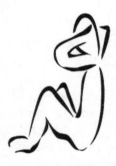

Exercise can be a wonderful thing. It can have remarkable benefits for our health, both physical and mental, and can greatly improve our sense of well-being. However, despite all the benefits of regular exercise many Irish men do not take enough exercise to stay healthy. And you know what? Some doctors are no exception here either. Despite all the medical evidence about the health benefits of exercise, some doctors either conveniently ignore this information or live in denial. As the proverb goes, 'Do as I say and not as I do.' Personally, I can't imagine trying to deal with the challenges of modern healthcare without the stress-busting benefits of regular exercise. What's more, it can be great fun staying in good shape.

Why Don't We Exercise?

Maybe we think we are too busy. The pace of modern life, combined with often long commutes to and from work, can squeeze our most precious commodity – time. Yet time is always made available for anything urgent that crops up in our lives, while things that are invaluable to our long-term health, such as regular exercise, can often be omitted, forgotten or put on the long finger.

Perhaps we are planning on taking more exercise at some time in the future when we are more organised and less busy. Unfortunately for many of us the reality is that that day never comes. Look at the shocking rates of heart disease and the explosion of obesity-related conditions, such as diabetes, amongst Irish men and you will quickly realise that procrastination won't get you anywhere. The key to success in life is to take action and just 30 minutes of moderate exercise daily can have substantial health benefits. Men who exercise regularly in general have better health, fewer illnesses and live longer.

Why Is Exercise so Good for My Health?

Regular exercise can have tremendous benefits for our health, both physical and psychological. Regular rigorous exercise is best and walking for 30 to 45 minutes on most days of the week at a moderate pace will do the trick. The key is that to really enjoy the health benefits of exercise it must be regular. You can't store up the benefits of exercise; so a mad burst of activity once a week just won't do the trick. Also, it's never too late to start taking exercise, no matter how unfit you may be. They say every journey begins with a single step – take that first step today and make exercise part of a better, healthier you.

Physical Benefits

- Exercise strengthens the heart muscle, thereby reducing the risk of heart attack. It also helps reduce the risk factors like high blood pressure, being overweight and high cholesterol that can contribute to heart disease. If you already have heart disease then exercise can reduce your chance of having another heart attack.

- Regular exercise lowers blood pressure and reduces the risk of stroke.
- Exercise tends to thin the blood, making it less likely to clot.
- Exercise helps lower cholesterol levels and regular exercise raises the HDL (good) cholesterol level, lowers the LDL (bad) cholesterol level and also helps to lower the blood fat (triglycerides) level by helping your metabolism to burn fat (see Chapter 6).
- Exercise helps to stimulate the metabolism, not just during exercise but also for up to 36 hours afterwards, helping to burn up calories and fat.
- Exercise helps to burn sugar and fat, thereby reducing your weight, which helps to prevent obesity.
- Regular exercise reduces the risk of developing diabetes.
- In people with diabetes, regular exercise significantly reduces the risk of heart disease and some cancers.
- Exercise helps strengthen the muscles, helping to stabilise the body and protect against falls. Weight training is more effective than aerobic exercise for bone strengthening.
- Exercise can reduce the risk of developing bowel cancer.
- Exercise can help prevent fractures caused by thinning of the bones (osteoporosis).
- Exercise can also help your memory and brain functioning. This may protect against memory disorders such as Alzheimer's disease.
- Regular exercise helps protect men against erectile dysfunction.
- Exercise can boost the immune system.
- Exercise also helps protect against the ageing process itself. There can be a huge difference between your age as determined by your date of birth and your biological age.

Psychological Benefits

Regular exercise has been shown to be very good for our mental health. It helps in the production of serotonin, which is a brain chemical necessary for feeling well. Deficiency of serotonin is widely recognised to be associated with symptoms of flatness, anxiety and depression. These symptoms are prevalent in Irish men anyway, especially in the winter months. We can therefore use a regular exercise programme to improve our mood and self-esteem and help to combat anxiety or depression. Indeed, exercise can be a great stress buster and is probably one of nature's best natural antidepressants.

Regular exercise can help promote good restful sleep. However, it is best to avoid heavy exercise late at night as this can affect sleep quality.

The Overall Package

The health benefits of regular exercise can be dramatic. A stronger heart and a healthier, more finely-tuned body can help prevent heart disease, some cancers and many other conditions. A stronger mind, less stressed and more balanced, is more conducive to optimal mental well-being. The result overall is a healthier life and, on average, a longer one. Not bad for a commitment of only half an hour a day.

Is All Exercise the Same?

There are three main types of exercise and a good exercise programme should include elements of all three:

1. Aerobic exercise, such as walking, running and swimming. This form of exercise causes the heart to pump more blood and beat faster. Most of the health benefits from exercise are gained through aerobic exercise.

2. Strength training, for example, lifting weights. This type of exercise is particularly good for strengthening the muscles and bones, particularly in middle age. For optimal benefits, some strength training for about 15 minutes twice a week is recommended. This will help to keep the muscles and body strong. However, this type of exercise does not have the same overall health benefits as aerobic exercise.

3. Flexibility exercises such as stretching, yoga and Pilates. This type of exercise is very good for relaxation as well as preventing stiffness and injury. Some flexibility exercises should be a part of everyone's routine.

Aerobic Exercise

Aerobic exercise is exercise that causes the heart to beat faster, improving oxygen consumption in the body. We know that simple walking provides excellent health benefits, even at low intensity. However, the heart is a muscle and a pump that strengthens with more vigorous exercise, especially when the heart rate increases to a target heart rate. At this target heart rate the body is thought to be exercising at its optimum. This target heart rate is generally 70 to 80 per cent of your age-adjusted maximum heart rate, which is calculated by the following formula:

220 - your age (in years) = maximum heart rate

So, for example, a 40-year-old male's maximum heart rate is calculated accordingly:

Maximum heart rate = 220 - 40 = 180

His target heart rate for aerobic exercise purposes is 70 to 80 per cent of 180, giving a range from 126 to 144.

Checking your heart rate is a good way to ensure that you are exercising at your target heart rate and that you are not overdoing it.

Checking Your Own Pulse

It is very easy to check your own pulse, which can be felt at your wrist beside your thumb or at your neck under the side of your jaw. If you are unsure or not confident about this, your family doctor will be happy to assist you. By counting your pulse for 10 seconds and then multiplying the answer by six you will know what your heart rate is per minute. An average resting heart rate is about seventy beats per minute and men who are fitter have lower rates. Once you are comfortable checking your own pulse, you can then check it during exercise to see if you are at your target heart rate.

Weight or Strength Training

Weight training is very important for keeping our muscles and bones strong and healthy. As we get older, this becomes particularly important for upper body strength, which tends to naturally decline with age. Body-building is not the aim. Two 15-minute sessions spaced out during the week are ideal. Put the emphasis on doing comfortable repetitions of low weights rather than going for broke on the Olympic bar. Press-ups are an excellent exercise for upper body strength. As with other forms of exercise, it is important not to overdo it. Listen to your own body and know the difference between a little bit of exercise-induced stiffness and the soreness that can come from an injury.

Flexibility Exercises

Stretching should be an essential part of any exercise programme, as it helps to keep the body loose and prevent injury. Working on and improving flexibility is also an important part of any rehabilitation programme after an injury. Exercises to strengthen the lower back and stomach muscles, often called core stabilisation exercises, are now recognised as being very important in injury prevention.

Stretching is also a great way to relax and unwind. The best stretching routine is the one that works best for you. Your doctor or physiotherapist can help you plan a specific programme for your needs.

There is a much greater emphasis on incorporating a more holistic approach to healthcare today. This can be seen by the increasing popularity of yoga, Pilates and tai chi. Personally I have been impressed by some elderly patients who practise yoga, especially with regard to their degree of flexibility and suppleness. Don't assume that yoga and Pilates are for women only, men can get the same health benefits from these activities.

How Much Exercise is Enough?

We were born to exercise. Primitive man was a hunter and gatherer and may have run many miles on a daily basis, gathering berries and escaping the clutches of lions and other wild beasts. However, this hunter–gatherer role has diminished as society has modernised, and now modern man can often spend his day sitting at a desk, behind a wheel of a car or slouched in front of a computer or TV screen. Of course this doesn't describe all of us, but you get the picture. We need to be much more proactive about taking exercise. It is felt that we need at least 30 minutes of moderate exercise daily or on most days of the week, i.e. 210 minutes per week. This is what is needed to keep our hearts, bodies and minds healthy. Moderate exercise means that you should get warm, but you don't have to sweat.

Know Your Numbers

- 30 minutes/day on most days (at least 5 times per week) or
- 210 minutes/week of moderate exercise
- 45–60 minutes/day if overweight or at risk of obesity
- 60–90 minutes/day if obese
- 10,000 steps equates to 5 miles/8 kilometres

If you have been inactive then the following tips may apply.

Easy does it. Better to start with a 10- or 15-minute walk daily and build this up over a few weeks as your body gets used to it. Remember, taking exercise each day does not have to involve going to the gym. Simple measures can work to increase your activity levels on a daily basis. These may include:

- Parking your car further away from your office. This can give you a chance to get a 5- or 10-minute walk each way.
- Taking the stairs where possible instead of the elevator
- Going for a walk at lunch time
- Buying a pedometer (step counter). This is an inexpensive and fairly accurate gadget that can measure how many steps you take each day. It works by detecting the motion of the hips and is thought to be accurate to within 5 to 10 per cent. Try to aim for 10,000 steps per day when you are up and at it. This can be a very useful motivational tool to help increase your activity levels.

Keeping an exercise diary can be a useful way of tracking your progress in this area. By using a weekly planner you can schedule in days and times when you plan to take exercise. Reviewing this on a weekly basis can allow you to see how well you did over the previous week, whether you achieved your target and how you can improve in the following week. This weekly diary is a great way to monitor your progress in a wide range of health parameters, especially diet and exercise.

Walking is great exercise for almost everyone. It can be a good way to stay in shape and can also be quite sociable, if you walk with a partner or friend. Remember, life is not a dress rehearsal. Do not put off until tomorrow what you can do today.

The only rule about exercise is that there are no rules. To get the maximum health benefits from exercise this 'magic health pill' needs to be taken regularly, ideally on a daily basis, but at least four to five times a week. After that you are free to choose whatever works for you.

Can Exercise Be Harmful?

For most people, most of the time, exercise is very safe and only good for your health. By following the six sensible steps listed below you can minimise the risks of any health-related problems connected with exercise. Sudden death during exercise has received a lot of publicity recently. This is quite rare and more likely to occur when someone takes intense vigorous exercise after a period of inactivity, for example, a vigorous game of squash. Sudden Athletic Death Syndrome (SADS) appears to have become more prevalent in recent times and can tragically result in the loss of young life. The precise cause is unknown and is the subject of ongoing research. Sometimes it is caused by an irregularity of the heartbeat or thickening of the heart muscle (called cardiomyopathy). Screening for these conditions can sometimes lead to the early detection of possible future cardiac problems.

Six Sensible Steps for Safer Exercise:

1. Safety first. Have a medical check-up before you begin a moderately vigorous exercise programme. Your doctor can help you tailor your exercise programme to your specific requirements.
2. Listen to your body. Don't exercise if you have a high temperature or feel unwell. If you get short of breath or develop chest pain, dizziness or palpitations during exercise, stop and seek medical attention.
3. Start low and go slow. This is particularly important if you haven't been used to taking exercise. Build up gradually over a

few weeks both the intensity and duration of exercise, which gives your body a chance to get used to the new regime and minimises the risk of injury. Wear proper footwear.

4. Warm up and stretch before and particularly after exercise – this is very good for flexibility and helps to prevent stiffness and injury.

5. Don't eat for 2 hours before intense exercise.

6. Stay hydrated – remember to drink plenty of fluids. Keeping well hydrated before, during and after exercise is very important to prevent cramp and injury as well as helping to optimise performance and improve recovery afterwards. Remember, thirst is a very poor indicator of hydration and by the time you feel thirsty you may already be quite dehydrated.

Steps To Staying Hydrated

- Ensure your urine is clear in colour – urine that is yellowish or dark in colour suggests dehydration.
- Drink about a pint of water in the hour or so before exercise, especially if the exercise activity will last an hour or more.
- Drink about 150–200 mls every 15 minutes during demanding exercise, especially in hot weather.
- Afterwards, drink plenty of fluids, including those containing some salt and carbohydrate (isotonic sports drinks). Avoid alcohol prior to exercise and remember to rehydrate with water or sports drinks afterwards and before taking alcohol.

How Fit Are You?

The following questionnaire can give you a good idea of how active you already are and how much further you need to go to get into the 'zone' of better health.

General Practice Physical Activity Questionnaire

1. Please tell us the type and amount of physical activity involved in your work. Please tick one box that best corresponds with your present work from the following four possibilities:

Please tick one box only

a. I am not in employment (e.g. retired, retired for health reasons, unemployed, full-time carer, etc.). ☐

b. I spend most of my time at work sitting (such as in an office). ☐

c. I spend most of my time at work standing or walking. However, my work does not require much intense physical effort (e.g. shop assistant, hairdresser, security guard, childminder, etc.). ☐

d. My work involves definite physical effort, including handling of heavy objects and use of tools (e.g. plumber, electrician, carpenter, cleaner, hospital nurse, gardener, postal delivery workers, etc.). ☐

e. My work involves vigorous physical activity, including handling of very heavy objects (e.g. scaffolder, construction worker, refuse collector, etc.). ☐

2. During the last week, how many hours did you spend on each of the following activities?

Please answer whether you are in employment or not.

	None	Some but less than 1 hour	1 hour but less than 3 hours	3 hours or more
a. Physical exercise such as swimming, jogging, aerobics, football, tennis, gym workout, etc.	☐	☐	☐	☐

(Continued)

65

(Continued)

	None	Some but less than 1 hour	1 hour but less than 3 hours	3 hours or more
b. Cycling, including cycling to work and during leisure time	☐	☐		☐
c. Walking, including walking to work, shopping, for pleasure, etc.	☐	☐	☐	☐
d. Housework/Childcare	☐	☐	☐	☐
e. Gardening/DIY	☐	☐	☐	☐

Please tick one box only on each row

3. How would you describe your usual walking pace? Please tick one box only.

Slow pace (i.e. less than 3 mph) ☐   Steady average pace ☐

Brisk pace ☐   Fast pace (i.e. over 4 mph) ☐

Key

Inactive — Sedentary job and no recreational physical activity

Moderately inactive — Sedentary job and some but < 1 hour recreational physical activity per week OR Standing job and no recreational physical activity

Moderately active — Sedentary job and 1–2.9 hours recreational physical activity per week OR Physical job and no recreational physical activity OR Standing job and some but < 1 hour recreations physical activity per week

Active — Sedentary job and ≥ 3 hours recreational physical activity per week OR Standing job and 1–2.9 hours recreational physical activity per week OR Physical job and some but < 1 hour recreational physical activity per week OR Heavy manual job

Conclusion

The health benefits of exercise are now widely recognised and some doctors prescribe exercise to their patients instead of pills. It could be said that exercise is probably the closest thing there is to an anti-aging pill. This is the one pill you can prescribe for yourself every day with long-lasting health benefits. Try it for yourself. Every journey begins with that first step.

Exercise Diary

Day	Activity	Time Duration/Minutes
Monday	Brisk walk	40 minutes
Tuesday	Swim and light weights	30 minutes and 10 minutes
Wednesday	Walk	30 minutes
Thursday	Stretching exercises	20 minutes
Friday	Swim and light weights	30 minutes and 10 minutes
Saturday	Rest	—
Sunday	Long walk	60 minutes

Total exercise per week = 210 minutes

- Keeping a record of your exercise habits can help you see how much (or how little) exercise you are really taking over a week.
- It can help you to plan exercise as an important part of your schedule.
- By looking at your time in chunks of a week at a time, you can plan more effectively.
- An exercise diary can be a great motivational tool.

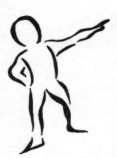

Key Points

- Regular exercise is essential for good long-term physical and mental well-being.
- No matter how unfit you are, it's never too late to start taking exercise and to start enjoying the health benefits.
- Make an exercise programme a priority for your better well-being.
- Set realistic, achievable goals.
- Stay positive.

5

A Good Heart

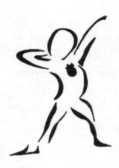 The human heart is an organ that is about the size of a closed fist and it is located in the chest behind the breast bone, in the middle and to the left. The heart is an amazing organ. It is basically a muscular pump designed to pump blood, firstly to the lungs where it gets oxygen, and then all around the body to the organs and muscles that need the oxygenated blood.

Vital Statistics

The heart beats and pumps on average seventy times per minute or over one hundred thousand times per day. This equates to over two and a half billion cycles over seventy years, and all this without maintenance. It is a truly remarkable pump and without comparison in engineering terms.

However, this heart muscle can become damaged. This damage mainly occurs if the small blood vessels supplying blood and oxygen to the heart itself become narrowed or blocked. Your heart is a muscle and like any other muscle in the body it needs oxygen, good nutrition and plenty of exercise to stay at its best. The plumbing of the heart muscle is provided by small arteries called the coronary arteries, which are wrapped around the heart muscle itself. There are three of these: the LCA (left coronary artery), the RCA (right coronary artery) and the circumflex artery. Narrowing of these arteries results in heart disease and sudden blockage can cause heart attack. The LCA is known as the 'widow-makers' artery' as blockage of this artery can result in sudden death.

Heart Disease – The Silent Killer

Perhaps the biggest problem with heart disease is that you may not know you have it. Narrowing of the coronary arteries can occur over many years without necessarily causing any symptoms. Indeed, men who get heart-related chest pain (called angina) may be the lucky ones in that they get an early warning that something is not right. The first symptom or sign of heart disease may be a heart attack or even sudden death. There is no doubt that early detection, and preferably prevention, of heart disease is much better than cure.

Risk Factors for Heart Disease

As an Irish male you are already at an increased risk of heart disease. Indeed, Irish men have some of the highest rates of heart disease in the world. This is largely because of the following risk factors:

- Our genetic makeup – there is no doubt that a family history is important for many conditions, including heart disease. Know your family history well and take appropriate action.
- Smoking – cigarette smoking approximately doubles your risk of heart attack. If you smoke, stop. The good news is that your risk of heart attack drops rapidly if you do stop.

- High blood pressure
- High cholesterol levels
- A 'Western diet' – typically a diet high in saturated fat
- Age – none of us can turn back the clock, but the risk of heart attack increases after the age of 40.
- Lack of exercise – the sedentary 'couch potato' lifestyle
- Diabetes
- High levels of stress/distress
- Heavy alcohol intake
- Obesity

Symptoms of Heart Disease

The main symptoms of heart disease are chest pain and tightness. As a muscle, the heart needs a good oxygen supply to keep pumping effectively. When there is narrowing of the coronary arteries there is less oxygen going to the heart muscle. This heart muscle can then develop cramp, just like any other muscle in the body. This heart cramp is known medically as angina. Initially, angina tends to come on when the heart is under extra pressure, for example, when exercising, such as climbing stairs or walking in cold weather, or when we are under stress. In other words, any situation where the heart has to work harder and therefore needs more oxygen can cause angina. Angina typically causes central-chest tightness and discomfort, often radiating upwards towards the jaw and sometimes down the left arm. It is often described as being like a tightness or pressure on the chest. An attack of angina is generally eased by rest.

Other symptoms of heart disease can include feeling short of breath when exercising, not being able to do as much as previously and getting tired easily. However, many people with heart disease have no symptoms at all until they have a heart attack.

Heart Attack

This is the biggest killer in Irish men. It is also known as myocardial infarction or coronary thrombosis. What happens is that one of the coronary arteries becomes completely blocked, causing severe cramp in the heart and causing the affected area of muscle to die if its blood supply is not restored relatively quickly. This can lead to serious irregularities of the heartbeat and the heart can stop completely. If the heart is not restarted within 3 minutes, either by resuscitation (CPR) or by the use of an external defibrillator, then irreversible brain and heart damage will occur.

Symptoms of a Heart Attack

Symptoms of a heart attack include a central crushing chest pain (like an elephant sitting on your chest), often radiating upwards to the neck and down either arm, more commonly the left arm, or down into your tummy area. This is often associated with profuse sweating, dizziness, shortness of breath, a sense of nausea or vomiting, and feeling acutely unwell. These symptoms are often compounded by an acute sense of fear or stress, which causes a massive adrenaline release to make the heart try to work even harder and harder, which makes the pain worse and worse. Clearly symptoms such as these need immediate medical attention. Early detection and treatment of heart attack can be life-saving. Clot-busting drugs have become available in recent years that can literally dissolve the blockage in your artery if given quickly enough.

Tests on Your Heart

For the Irish man all of this means you should be aware of your risk factors for heart disease and also understand the symptoms of heart disease and be able to take appropriate action. This means a regular check-up with your doctor, focusing on preventative health issues. A good chat with your doctor, along with some tests, will help give you a better understanding of your risks. Tests include examining your weight (body mass index), waist circumference, pulse and blood pressure, along with a cardiac examination and some blood tests, such as examining your lipid profile (for cholesterol and blood fat) and blood glucose levels (for risk or tendency to diabetes).

ECG Test

If your doctor suspects heart disease he may suggest some additional tests, which may include an ECG (electrocardiogram). This is an office-based test in which a number of stickers are placed on the chest wall and the electrical rhythm in the heart is recorded. This ECG test can be very useful in determining any strain on the heart or any heart irregularities. Many of these ECGs can now be analysed by computer.

An exercise ECG (stress test) can also be carried out. This is where you are put onto a treadmill and hooked up to an ECG while you exercise, walking at a slow pace initially and gradually building up until you are jogging. The heart rhythm and rate are recorded. If there are narrowings in the coronary arteries this will cause additional strain on the heart muscle as you exercise, which may show up on the ECG test. However, these tests are not black and white, and some cases of heart disease may remain undetected, even if these tests are normal.

Echocardiogram

An echocardiogram (echo) is an ultrasound scan of the heart muscle used to look at how well the heart muscle and heart valves are working. It can be a very useful test when heart problems are suspected. Sometimes an echo can detect congenital abnormalities such as thickening of the heart muscle wall, which can be associated with an increased risk of sudden cardiac death. An example of such a condition is HOCM (hypertrophic obstructive cardiomyopathy).

<u>Angiogram</u>

An angiogram is another test that can be done to look at the coronary arteries. In this test a thin flexible tube known as a catheter is guided from a leg artery up into the coronary arteries in the heart. Dye is then injected into the catheter and repeated x-ray pictures are taken as the dye flows through the heart. This allows any narrowing or tiny blockages in the blood vessels to show up.

More recent advanced scanning technology can also allow detailed images of the heart to be taken, which can give a good indication of blockages and damaged arteries.

Treatments for Heart Disease

<u>Angioplasty</u>

This is an effective procedure used to widen narrowed arteries in the heart. Once an angiogram has located the narrowed part of the coronary artery, a thin expandable balloon can be guided over a wire to the affected area. This balloon tip can then be inflated and so expands the artery by stretching the artery open. This can significantly reduce the blockage in the artery. Major complications from this procedure are uncommon. However, sometimes the artery narrows again in the six months after angioplasty. This is known as 'restenosis' and may need further treatment.

<u>Stent Procedure</u>

This is where a small tube is left in the narrowed artery after angioplasty. This is like a support structure for the artery. It keeps the narrowed part of the artery open and thereby improves the blood supply to the heart muscle. This has been a major advance in the treatment of heart disease. Newer stents have been devised that are coated with drugs to thin the blood and can help prevent reclosure at the stent site.

<u>Heart Bypass Surgery</u>

This is a type of heart surgery known as coronary artery bypass grafting (CABG) by which blood is re-routed around blocked arteries by creating bypasses around them with veins taken from other parts of the body, usually the legs. This procedure is less often performed now due to the newer innovations in the treatment of narrowed or blocked arteries, such as angioplasty and stents, as well as better medical management of heart-related problems.

What Can I Do to Prevent Heart Disease?

Prevention is better than cure and we know that heart disease is a largely preventable condition. You can't change your age or your genetic makeup and family history. However, you can make dramatic improvements to your heart health and add years to your life expectancy and quality of life by taking action and making positive changes. And it is never too late to make those positive changes, even if you have several risk factors for heart disease and even if you have heart disease already.

- If you smoke, stop smoking! Smoking twenty cigarettes a day doubles your risk of heart attack because smoking makes the blood thicker, enabling it to clot more easily. Smoking cigarettes also causes carbon monoxide, which blocks oxygen from getting to the muscles, to enter the bloodstream. Smoking destroys Vitamin C, which helps protect the heart, and, most importantly, it causes damage to the lining of the blood vessels, thus facilitating clotting and blockages.

- Have a regular check-up and make sure your blood pressure is well controlled at 120/80.
- Keep your total cholesterol level under 5, your LDL (bad) cholesterol level under 3 and your HDL (good) cholesterol level over 1 (see Chapter 6 for an explanation of the different types of cholesterol).
- Eat a heart-healthy diet, focusing on fruit and vegetables, wholegrains, plenty of fibre, oats, oily fish, and eating plenty of foods rich in antioxidants (mainly fruit and vegetables, seeds and pulses). Reduce your dietary salt intake and minimise your saturated fat intake.
- Develop an active lifestyle and exercise regularly – at least 210 minutes a week (30 minutes a day).
- Monitor your stress levels – look at your work–life balance, learn to de-stress and give yourself enough down time.
- Moderate your alcohol intake – less is more. For most people, who are otherwise not addicted or allergic to alcohol, 1 or 2 units of alcohol per day may have a cardio-protective effect. This is partly due to the benefits of alcohol on HDL cholesterol as well helping the blood to clot. However, more than two drinks per day increases your risk of heart disease. Be aware of your safe limits.

<u>What about Supplements to Prevent Heart Disease?</u>

Folic acid and the B vitamins can lower homocysteine levels, which tend to be high in Celtic males. Homocysteine is an amino acid implicated in the hardening of the arteries and high levels are a factor in heart disease. Folic acid, either taken through diet or in supplementary form, lowers homocysteine levels and can be a useful addition in the fight against heart disease and stroke. In addition, niacin

(Vitamin B₃) is very helpful at raising HDL (good) cholesterol levels. This is discussed further in Chapter 6.

Omega-3 fish oil, particularly that found in cold water fish (such as salmon, tuna and sardines) or else in supplement form, is beneficial for the heart. Again this is discussed in Chapter 6.

Coenzyme Q is produced by the human body and is necessary for the basic working of cells. It is thought that coenzyme Q levels can be low in patients with some chronic diseases, such as heart conditions and high blood pressure. Some prescription drugs, such as statins for cholesterol, may also lower coenzyme Q levels. Therefore a coenzyme Q supplement may reduce some of the potential side effects of statin treatment for raised cholesterol and may also help to lower blood pressure. This area is the subject of ongoing research.

What About Aspirin?

Aspirin can prevent clotting occurring at the site of narrowed arteries by thinning the blood. Because platelets (the cells in the blood that are involved in blood clotting) are made on a continuous basis by the bone marrow, aspirin must be taken on a regular basis, either daily or every second day, to have its maximum effect.

If you have already suffered a heart attack or have established heart disease then taking low-dose aspirin has an important role in preventing further heart attack or further heart damage. Low doses of aspirin (between 75mg and 300mg per day) will produce this vital benefit. For many men who do not already have heart disease, taking a low-dose aspirin daily or on alternate days may have health benefits in terms of reducing your risk of heart attack. This blood-thinning ability of aspirin is generally better in men over fifty.

Because aspirin is a blood thinner it can help men who have peripheral artery disease (PAD) or damage to the circulation in their legs. Aspirin can also help prevent the most common type of stroke, i.e. that form of stroke caused by a blood clot in the brain. However, because aspirin thins the blood it does increase the risk of the rarer hemorrhagic stroke, which is brain damage caused by a bleed into the brain itself. Aspirin may also have some benefit in terms of preventing colon (bowel) cancer. This is an area of ongoing research.

However, despite the fact that it is widely available as an over-the-counter medicine, this does not mean that aspirin is always safe. In some people it can cause serious side effects; the most common is bleeding, especially bleeding after injury. Because of this you should always stop your aspirin at least a week before elective surgery. Bleeding from the stomach lining can cause stomach or duodenal ulcers. Aspirin can also affect the kidneys, particularly in elderly people. Some people can have allergies to aspirin and must avoid it.

There are pros and cons to taking aspirin, just like every other drug. Ultimately the decision will rest with you, in consultation with your doctor.

Blood Pressure – The Silent Killer

What Is Blood Pressure?

Blood pressure is simply the pressure of blood in the tubes as it is brought around the body. It is measured in millimetres of mercury (mmHg) and is quoted as two separate figures, e.g. 120/80. The upper figure is known as the systolic blood pressure. This is the pressure of blood in the tubes when the heart beats and contracts, causing blood to be squeezed and pumped from the heart to all parts of the body. The second figure is known as the diastolic figure or resting blood pressure. This is the pressure in the tubes when the heart relaxes after beating. This cycle of beat, relax, beat, relax repeats itself continuously. Normal blood pressure varies over a 24-hour period. Exercise will cause blood pressure to temporarily go up, as higher pressure is needed to vigorously pump blood into exercising muscles that need more oxygen. When we are under stress the 'flight or fight' response kicks in, whereby hormones such as cortisol and adrenaline are released from the adrenal glands (small glands that sit on top of the kidneys). The net effect of these hormones is to cause blood pressure to go up. Conversely, when we are sleeping at night-time blood pressure is usually lower as our bodies rest and relax.

What Is High Blood Pressure?

High blood pressure is when your blood pressure reading is higher than what is considered acceptable for good health. It may be indicated by a raised systolic blood pressure reading, a raised diastolic blood pressure reading, or both. As blood pressure readings can vary throughout the day, a once-off raised reading is not of any major significance. However, repeated raised blood pressure readings, ideally averaged over a 24-hour period using a 24-hour blood pressure monitor, can easily indicate high blood pressure.

How Common Is It?

High blood pressure is very common and is one of the leading risk factors for heart disease and stroke in the Western world. It can affect up to one in every four middle-aged Irish men and about one in every two Irish men aged over 65.

High blood pressure is one of those medical conditions that follows a rule known as 'the rule of halves'. This means that about half of all people with high blood pressure remain undiagnosed and do not know they have it. This includes a lot of Irish men who haven't been to the doctor for years because they 'feel fine'. About half of those diagnosed are not treated and only about half of those who get treatment have their treatment properly controlled according to best practice guidelines. Therefore, as few as one in eight people with high blood pressure have their condition properly diagnosed, treated and controlled. There are many complex reasons why this rule of halves exists; these include the reluctance amongst Irish men to go to the doctor, the lack of emphasis on prevention in healthcare and the resistance of many men to taking medication when they don't feel sick.

How Do I Know If I Have High Blood Pressure?

High blood pressure is often known as a silent disease because there may be no symptoms whatsoever. A person with high blood pressure feels well, looks well and rarely has any symptoms. Indeed, unless a man goes for a check-up and has his blood pressure checked, he may never know he has high blood pressure until it is too late.

If your blood pressure reading is up then several readings on different occasions are needed to confirm that your blood pressure is indeed elevated. Some men suffer from what is known as the 'white-coat effect', whereby anxiety due to unease or insecurity when going to the doctor can cause the blood pressure to temporarily go up. Taking readings on different occasions can sometimes help overcome this white-coat effect. However, the most accurate way to diagnose high blood pressure now is to use a 24-hour blood pressure monitor. This is where a cuff attached to a small computerised monitor is wrapped around your arm and you carry on with your normal business for 24 hours, after which the cuff is removed and the data is printed out on a computer. This monitor checks your blood pressure at 30-minute intervals over the entire 24-hour period. A detailed graph can then be printed out showing your overall average blood pressure as well as your average day-time and night-time readings and what percentage of each are above normal.

What Causes High Blood Pressure?

The exact cause of high blood pressure is unknown. There is often no single cause and it is thought to be due to a combination of many different factors. High blood pressure often runs in families. It is not due to being nervous or highly strung. Firstly, the ageing process itself can cause the blood vessels to become less elastic and flexible and more hard or rigid. This loss of elasticity in the blood vessel walls can cause the pressure of blood going through them to go up. It is not ageing per se but rather ageing of the blood vessels that causes this hardening and resultant increase in pressure. This hardening of the blood vessels is often caused by cigarette smoking and the high-saturated-fat, high-salt diet so prevalent in the Western world.

Cigarette smoking can damage the lining of the blood vessels, causing them to narrow over time. This will make the pressure of blood going through these narrow tubes go up, as the heart has to pump harder to push the blood through a narrow space.

High cholesterol and blood fat (triglycerides) levels, caused either by a high-saturated-fat diet or by genetic factors, can lead to the formation of cholesterol plaques on the inside of the blood vessels, which causes the tubes to narrow. This is a condition known as atherosclerosis.

A diet rich in salt can also cause blood pressure to go up as sodium causes fluid retention and also affects the complex hormonal pathways that regulate blood pressure.

Obesity or carrying excess weight is also associated with an increased risk of high blood pressure. A simple analogy is that, for every extra pound of fat, there is approximately an extra mile of tiny blood vessels supplying blood to that pound of fat. So suppose you are 3 stone overweight, that means every time your heart beats it has to pump blood an extra 42 miles. In that context it is easy to see how pressure goes up, as the heart has to work harder to bring oxygen to that extra fat. While this analogy is not totally accurate, it gets the message across.

Genetic factors are obviously important in the development of high blood pressure. If there is a history of high blood pressure in your family, you need to pay extra attention to your own risk of developing high blood pressure in the future.

High blood pressure is also very common in people with diabetes, as diabetes can lead to hardening of the arteries. Stress is also recognised as a potential cause of raised blood pressure. The fight or flight response is a normal reaction in the body to feeling under stress. However, if you are under chronic long-term stress, then the long-term effect of hormones like cortisol and adrenaline on the system can result in high blood pressure. More rarely, raised blood pressure can be caused by hormonal conditions like Cushing's syndrome and other disorders of the adrenal glands.

What Are the Complications of Raised Blood Pressure?

For many years raised blood pressure may cause no symptoms. Occasionally, raised blood pressure can be associated with headaches and nose bleeds, but usually only when the blood pressure is very high. However, high blood pressure makes the heart and arteries work harder, causing damage over the years. This can lead to a heart attack or stroke at an early age. Fortunately, treatment can reverse most of these effects.

However, raised blood pressure can have devastating consequences by putting extra strain on the system over a long period of time. These complications can include blindness, kidney damage, heart attacks and mini-strokes, as well as full-blown strokes. These complications can come on suddenly with devastating effects.

High blood pressure is, along with cigarette smoking, the most important risk factor for the development of heart disease and stroke. Other risk factors for the development of heart disease and stroke include family history, raised cholesterol and blood fat levels, obesity, lack of exercise, excess alcohol and a diet high in saturated fat and salt. The important thing to note about these risk factors is that they are synergistic rather than additive. This means that they multiply together rather than add together. In other words, if you have three of these risk factors your risk of heart attack or stoke may be many times higher than if you just have two.

Benefits of Treating Raised Blood Pressure

Obviously prevention is better than cure. The aim in detecting and treating raised blood pressure is to bring the pressure back down to normal so as to prevent any long-term strain on the heart or blood vessels, thereby helping to prevent heart disease and stroke. If you have been prescribed medication for high blood pressure, you will usually have to take it for the rest of your life. If you stop the medication your blood pressure will tend to go up again. The good news is that this medication can prevent early ageing of the blood vessels and prevent any additional strain on the heart. There is good evidence that lowering your blood pressure, if it is raised, can significantly reduce your relative risk of both heart attack and stroke.

Can I Stop My Blood Pressure Tablets Once My Blood Pressure Is Back Down to Normal?

No, unfortunately. The decision to treat raised blood pressure is an important one as the treatment is usually lifelong. This is because, if you stop taking the blood pressure tablets, then your blood pressure will usually start to climb up again. Therefore it is very important that the diagnosis is made correctly and that the decision to treat it is a shared one between you and your doctor. By fully understanding the implications of the decision to treat high blood pressure in terms of the benefits of doing so as well as the risks and consequences of not treating your high blood pressure, you are then in a better position to weigh up the benefits of long-term treatment.

What About Changing My Lifestyle?

Certainly a heart-healthy lifestyle is conducive to good heart health and will help your blood pressure. If your blood pressure is only mildly elevated, then it may make sense to try a heart-healthy lifestyle for a period of three to six months, to see if your blood pressure benefits. If you are successful, you may avoid having to take long-term pressure treatment. A heart-healthy lifestyle would naturally include the following:

- Stopping smoking
- If you are overweight, losing weight – studies have shown that by losing 10 per cent of your body weight (if you are over-weight) you can reduce your blood pressure by ten mmHg
- Watching your alcohol intake – keep within the recommended limits for men of 21 units per week. Remember, less is more
- Regular exercise
- Eating a heart-healthy diet:
  - ○ eat plenty of fresh fruit and vegetables
  - ○ use fat-free or low-fat milk and dairy products
  - ○ switch to wholegrain cereal
  - ○ eat oily fish at least once or twice a week
  - ○ eat poultry and nuts
  - ○ eat foods that are rich in potassium, calcium and magnesium
  - ○ cut out trans-fats, saturated fat and cholesterol and reduce your total fat intake
  - ○ reduce red meat consumption to once a week or less
  - ○ cut out sweets and sources of added sugar
  - ○ minimise your salt intake – this in effect means avoiding processed foods, which tend to be high in salt.

Stroke

A stroke can also be called a brain attack. It is like a heart attack except that it is the brain that is affected. The blood supply to the brain is interrupted and cut off. This causes nerve cells in that part of the brain to die, which affects the body functions controlled by those brain cells. This is the often devastating consequence of stroke. Stroke is a common cause of death among Irish men.

What Causes a Stroke?

Strokes have two underlying causes: either a blockage of a brain artery or a bleed from an artery in the brain. Most strokes are caused by a blockage in one of the brain arteries as a result of the same risk factors and processes that cause heart disease, i.e. smoking, high cholesterol, high blood pressure, etc. Less commonly, strokes are caused by a rupture in a brain blood vessel, which causes bleeding into the brain tissue itself. This is often caused by high blood pressure or a brain aneurysm. An aneurysm is a weak area or bubble on a blood vessel that can be like a time bomb waiting to go off. Some people are born with aneurysms and sometimes they develop as a result of high blood pressure or hardening of the arteries.

What Are the Symptoms of Stroke?

As the name suggests, stroke is like a bolt of lightening, and can bring on sudden death. Symptoms include weakness or paralysis down one side of the body (face, arms or legs), numbness or loss of sensation in the face or limbs, and loss of bladder control, speech or vision. Other symptoms can include weakness, difficulty swallowing, face drooping to one side, dizziness, loss of balance, severe headache, difficulty speaking or understanding simple statements, and loss of vision, especially in one eye. There is potential for a certain amount of recovery in the first few weeks after a stroke, which is why expert rehabilitation with a range of different health professionals is so important.

What Type of Man Is at Risk of Stroke?

- Older men – two-thirds of strokes occur in people aged over 65.
- Those with a history of heart disease, previous stroke or mini-stroke
- Men with risk factors such as high blood pressure, high cholesterol, obesity and lack of exercise, smokers and heavy drinkers
- Those with an irregular heartbeat, called atrial fibrillation, which increases the chances of clots in the system
- Men with a high red blood cell count, as thicker blood is more likely to clot
- Men with a family history of stroke

Prevention of Stroke

Just like heart disease, you can reduce your chances of getting a stroke by making certain changes in your lifestyle, especially by not smoking and controlling high blood pressure. If you have high cholesterol, lowering your cholesterol levels may also reduce your risk. Your doctor may tell you to change your lifestyle as well as prescribing medication to lower your blood pressure or cholesterol. Aspirin or warfarin is often used to prevent clotting and reduce the risk of stroke.

Mini-Strokes

These are also known as transient ischemic attacks or TIAs, brought on when an artery in the brain becomes temporarily blocked. This can cause symptoms similar to a stroke but the symptoms disappear without any permanent damage within 24 hours. This is the key difference between a TIA and a stroke. However a TIA is a warning sign that you are at much greater risk of a stroke in the future. Therefore it is an early warning sign that you need to sit up and take notice of your health, and work with your doctor to do all that can be done to prevent a stroke later on.

Abdominal Aortic Aneurysms (AAA)

The aorta is the main blood vessel that comes from the heart and brings blood to the body. When it leaves the heart it initially goes upwards and then curves down through the tummy area to bring blood to the lower body and legs. Damage to the wall and lining of the aorta can cause it to weaken and bulge like a small bubble, creating an aneurysm. When an aneurysm develops on the aorta in the abdominal area it is known as an abdominal aortic aneurysm (AAA). This condition is more common in men, particularly middle-aged and elderly men.

What Causes AAA?

Cigarette smoking greatly increases the chance of getting an AAA and raised cholesterol and blood pressure levels, along with obesity, are also risk factors. Also, if there is a family history of the condition then your chances of getting it are much increased. The ageing process itself, particularly ageing of the blood vessels, can also play an important role.

Diagnosis

Most men with an AAA have no symptoms. Sometimes it can cause bellyache or backache. It may be possible to feel a large aneurysm in the tummy area as a pulsating or throbbing swelling. The most reliable and accurate way to diagnose an AAA is by a simple ultrasound scan. So if you have any of the risk factors, discuss the benefits of a screening ultrasound scan for an AAA. If one is detected then you will need to see a vascular specialist to determine whether it needs to be surgically repaired. Once an aneurysm has formed it will not go away on its own, so most aneurysms eventually need surgery. The main complication of an aneurysm is that it can eventually rupture or burst, with often fatal consequences. In this respect, an aneurysm can be a time bomb.

Treatment Options

A watch-and-wait approach with regular follow-up assessments is often advised for small aneurysms with no symptoms. In general terms, the risk of an AAA rupturing or bursting is related to its size. Small aneurysms (less than 5 centimetres in diameter) have a very low risk of rupture, whereas larger aneurysms have an increased risk. However, if it enlarges beyond 5 centimetres, surgery is required. The surgical repair of an AAA is generally a big operation with a risk of serious complications. The weakened aorta is replaced with a polyester tube or graft and stitched into place. This graft is permanent and will last for many years.

Recently, new breakthroughs in minimally invasive surgery can allow the aneurysm to be fixed from the inside out by making small incisions in the groin; thus, major incisions in the chest wall can often be avoided. Aortic aneurysms that have ruptured can be repaired with emergency surgery but the mortality rate from a ruptured aneurysm is high.

Peripheral Arterial Disease (PAD)

Atherosclerosis is a disease process in which arteries that bring blood to various parts of the body become damaged, resulting in narrowed arteries and potential blockages. When atherosclerosis affects the heart it makes the coronary arteries narrow, causing angina and heart attack; when it affects the brain it can cause TIAs (mini strokes) and stroke; when it affects the aorta it can cause an aneurysm (AAA); and when atherosclerosis affects the legs it causes Peripheral Arterial Disease (PAD). This can result in progressive narrowing of the arteries in the legs, leading to potential blockages and eventually possible gangrene, which would lead to amputation.

PAD does not get as much attention as heart disease or stroke and yet it is a very common and often under-diagnosed medical condition. It is thought to affect about one in every four Irish men over the age of seventy-five.

What Are the Risk Factors for PAD?

The risk factors for PAD are the same ones that damage the circulation elsewhere in the body, including the risk factors for heart disease and stroke. They include:

- Cigarette smoking
- Diabetes
- High cholesterol levels
- High blood pressure
- Obesity
- Lack of exercise
- Stress
- Family history

What Are the Symptoms?

Like other forms of atherosclerosis, PAD can be a silent condition with no symptoms for many years. The earliest symptom tends to be pain or cramping in the leg, which comes on with exercise. Classically, this pain or cramp disappears within a few minutes of resting. The symptom pattern is very variable. With more severe blockages, pain can also occur in the foot when resting, particularly at night-time.

How Is PAD Diagnosed?

Your doctor can examine your legs and assess the pulses in your feet. He can also look for other evidence of PAD such as loss of hair on the toes, skin changes (with the skin becoming pale and shiny) and loss of colour in the leg when it is elevated.

A simple test called the Ankle Brachial Pressure Index (ABI) can determine not only whether PAD is present but can also give a good estimate of its severity. The ABI test is simply a ratio of the blood pressure in your arm measured in the normal way, compared to the blood pressure in your leg measured using an ultrasound probe. The table below shows the scoring system that is used.

The ABI Scoring System for Peripheral Arterial Disease (PAD)

ABI	Severity of Blockages
0.9 or higher	None
0.7–0.89	Mild
0.5–0.69	Moderate
Below 0.5	Severe
Below 0.15	Threat of amputation

More detailed tests can be done for cases that may benefit from surgical intervention. These include scans and angiography, where dye is injected into the arteries to assess the extent of the blockages.

How Is PAD Treated?

Obviously, the first line of treatment is to eliminate any known risk factors. This includes stopping smoking, optimising your blood pressure, cholesterol and blood sugar levels, taking plenty of aerobic exercise, keeping your weight down and minimising stress. A good exercise programme can have amazing benefits on muscles because it can allow new blood vessels to form and sometimes create new little ring roads around blocked arteries. Exercise can also allow muscles to use oxygen more effectively, which makes them more efficient.

Medication has a limited role to play in patients with PAD. Plavix and aspirin are often used for people with established PAD because of their blood thinning and anti-clotting abilities. Alternative treatments that have been used include garlic and *Ginkgo biloba*, which are thought to have some circulation-enhancing benefits.

In more severe cases, blocked arteries can be unblocked by angioplasty and sometimes severe blockages are by-passed. Unfortunately, reblockage of the affected arteries can occur. As with many other conditions, prevention is better than cure. However, with meticulous attention to the risk factors, combined with a healthy lifestyle and vigorous exercise programme, the symptoms of PAD can often be kept under control and improved over time.

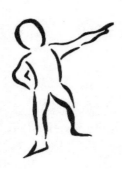

Key Points

- Heart disease and stroke are the number one causes of death and premature illness in Irish men.
- High blood pressure is very common in Irish men and is a major risk factor for heart disease and stroke.
- High blood pressure often has no symptoms; it is 'the silent killer'.
- Atherosclerosis is a disease process that damages the circulation and can affect the heart, brain, aorta and legs, causing heart disease, stroke, aneurysms and blocked arteries.

- We can't change our genes but many of the risk factors for atherosclerosis can be controlled – these include cigarette smoking, high blood pressure, diabetes, high cholesterol, stress, obesity and lack of exercise.
- Narrowing of the blood vessels in the legs (PAD) and aneurysm of the aorta (AAA) are both common in ageing men.
- Know your numbers – you should get your blood pressure and cholesterol checked regularly.
- High blood pressure, high cholesterol and many of the risk factors for heart disease, stroke and atherosclerosis can be very successfully treated, but only if you are aware that you have them.
- Prevention is better than cure.

6

Conquer Your Cholesterol

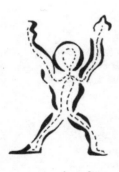

Cholesterol is mainstream news these days. Take a walk through any supermarket isle and you will be bombarded with signs for low-cholesterol and cholesterol-free products. Advertisements abound for dairy spreads that claim to lower your cholesterol. Pharmaceutical companies advertise cholesterol-lowering medication and its benefits. In some countries, such as the UK, this medication (statins) can now be purchased straight over the counter in pharmacies without a doctor's prescription.

You probably already know that cholesterol has something to do with heart disease. Heart disease is the biggest cause of death in Ireland for men, and one of the best ways to prevent heart disease is to keep your cholesterol at a healthy level. But, like many people, you may be confused about cholesterol, all the different fats you eat, what happens to them in your body and how they affect your heart. So what is the story with cholesterol? Why is it important? And what should you do about it?

What Is Cholesterol?

Cholesterol is a soft fatty-like substance that, in healthy amounts, is used by the body for normal cell function. You need a certain amount of cholesterol for all the cells in your body to work properly and to produce important hormones. Some of the cholesterol in our systems is made in the liver and we get the rest from our diets. Food rich in cholesterol and saturated fat will increase the amount of cholesterol in our systems.

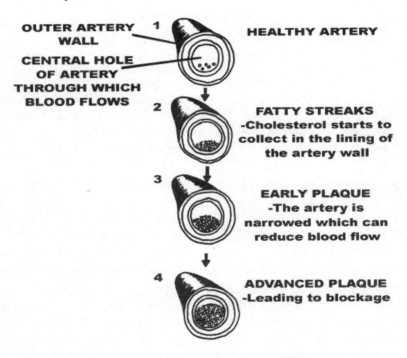

OUTER ARTERY WALL

CENTRAL HOLE OF ARTERY THROUGH WHICH BLOOD FLOWS

1 **HEALTHY ARTERY**

2 **FATTY STREAKS** -Cholesterol starts to collect in the lining of the artery wall

3 **EARLY PLAQUE** -The artery is narrowed which can reduce blood flow

4 **ADVANCED PLAQUE** -Leading to blockage

THE EFFECT OF CHOLESTEROL BUILD UP AND PLAQUE FORMATION

The problem is that, over time, excess cholesterol in the blood vessels can cause the cholesterol to stick to the walls of the blood vessels, leading to the development of fatty plaques (see diagram on page 94). These plaques can then cause narrowing of the blood vessels and eventually lead to heart disease or stroke.

In this context, it is worth knowing what the normal values of these types of cholesterol are. These are shown in the table below. There are two main types of cholesterol: LDL and HDL.

Know Your Numbers

Total cholesterol	Should be less than 5
LDL cholesterol (bad cholesterol)	Should be less than 3 or less than 2.5 if you are diabetic or if you already have heart disease, including heart attack, bypass or angioplasty. Some experts now say to keep LDL under 2.
HDL cholesterol (good cholesterol)	Should be greater than 1
Triglycerides (blood fat)	Should be less than 1.6

LDL Cholesterol

Firstly, the bad guy: LDL cholesterol. This is the bad cholesterol, which I call 'lousy' cholesterol. The less LDL or lousy cholesterol you have the better. This figure should be less than 3 millimoles/litre (less than 2.5 mmol/litre if you are diabetic or already have heart disease).

LDL cholesterol comes from two separate sources. Firstly, as most of us know, we get LDL cholesterol in our diets. Particular sources of LDL cholesterol include fried foods and stodgy carbohydrates. Secondly, LDL cholesterol is made in the liver and some people simply make too much LDL cholesterol. Therefore, even if you eat a very healthy diet, it is still possible to have high total and high LDL cholesterol levels.

What Do Raised LDL Cholesterol Levels Do To Me?

LDL cholesterol travels from the liver through the arteries to other parts of the body. Over time, raised LDL cholesterol levels can allow it to stick to the inner lining of your arteries or blood vessels, causing narrowing, hardening and ultimately blockage of the fine blood vessels that bring blood around the body to vital organs like the heart and the brain. Imagine sticky goo like sticky toffee pudding: this is just what LDL cholesterol is like, sticking to the walls of the blood vessels. This process of narrowing and hardening, known as atherosclerosis, occurs over many years. Raised cholesterol can be a silent condition, with no symptoms whatsoever, until one of the tubes blocks over and results in a heart attack or a stroke. High levels of LDL cholesterol increase your risk of heart disease.

Dietary Sources of LDL Cholesterol

Saturated fats can raise your LDL cholesterol levels and you find saturated fats in foods like butter, hard margarine, lard, cream, cheese, fatty meat, cakes, biscuits and chocolates. Processed foods are usually high in saturated fats.

Hydrogenated fats or trans-fats also raise the level of LDL cholesterol as well as accelerating the rate of artery blockage. Recently it has been shown that starchy carbohydrates can also increase your LDL cholesterol level. Examples of starchy carbohydrates include white bread, biscuits, cakes and many cereals (excluding oat-based cereals).

How Can I Lower My LDL Cholesterol Level?

There are a number of things you can do to help reduce your LDL cholesterol levels. Start off by having a good look at your diet.

Keeping a diary of everything you eat over a seven-day period, or at least over a weekend and one or two weekdays, can give you an ideal opportunity to look at not only what you eat but also when and why. This might throw up a few surprises for you. Cutting down significantly on starchy carbohydrates like white bread, biscuits and cakes and also on fries is a good place to start. It is useful to focus on positive changes that you are likely to stick to rather than being negative and saying 'I can't have this' and 'I can't have that.' Therefore, I would encourage you to think about heart-healthy options where possible:

- Eating oat-based cereals such as porridge seems to be very good for cholesterol because oats appear to bind to LDL cholesterol in the gut, thereby helping its removal from the bloodstream.
- Cut back on red meat intake significantly. Switch to lean white meat such as chicken instead. Avoid the skin of the chicken as it is high in cholesterol.
- Throw away the frying pan.
- Eat less saturated fat. Choose low-fat dairy products and low-fat spreads made from sunflower or olive oil.
- Eating cold water fish, or any fish for that matter, instead of meat may lower cholesterol and heart disease risk simply by reducing the amount of saturated fat in your diet. Eating oily fish such as salmon, mackerel, tuna and sardines several times a week is very good for heart health because these are rich in omega-3 fish oil. Other good sources of omega-3 include flaxseed, walnuts, soybeans and canola oil.
- Polyunsaturated and monounsaturated fats are unsaturated fats that can help lower the amount of LDL cholesterol in your blood and reduce your chances of getting heart disease. They are found in most pure vegetable oils and in the margarine spreads made from these oils. Examples include sunflower, olive and

rapeseed oils. Polyunsaturated fats are also found in oily fish such as salmon, sardines and mackerel.

- Eating lots of soluble fibre, wholegrain breads and pasta, and lots of fruit and vegetables is beneficial.
- Eggs in moderation are fine. While egg yolk is actually very high in cholesterol, it does not appear to contribute significantly to our blood cholesterol levels. As well as being rich in protein, eggs also have useful vitamins and minerals.
- If you are overweight, meaning your body mass index is greater than 25, then weight reduction can often improve LDL levels.
- Regular exercise is helpful, not only in terms of heart health and weight control, but also in helping to stabilise blood sugar levels, thereby preventing excess LDL production.
- Antioxidants are substances that are thought to prevent hardening of cholesterol to the blood vessel wall by reducing cholesterol's stickiness, tendency to clot and ability to damage the blood vessel wall. Antioxidants are also thought to play a role in cancer prevention. Fresh fruit and vegetables are considered to be excellent sources of antioxidants. Examples of antioxidants include Vitamins A, C and E, selenium and coenzyme Q. However, while some research has suggested that vitamins with antioxidant properties (such as beta carotene and Vitamins C and E) can lower the risk for heart disease, the evidence is, at best, conflicting. The best advice at present is simply to eat a diet rich in the fruits and vegetables that provide these vitamins, such as citrus fruit, broccoli and tomatoes. Green tea has a high level of antioxidants known as flavinoids and may have some beneficial effects.
- Folic acid also appears to be helpful in preventing hardening of the arteries by lowering homocysteine levels. Homocysteine is a

substance that is found in high levels in Celtic men. Some of the
B vitamins also seem to help lower homocysteine levels.

- If you smoke, you should stop. Smoking with high cholesterol is
like throwing petrol on a fire. Smoking damages the lining of the
small blood vessels, allowing cholesterol to stick to the damaged
blood vessel walls and thereby promoting the rapid development
of multiple blockages throughout the circulatory system.

- Garlic is a popular folk remedy for many health conditions and
some studies have shown a beneficial effect on cholesterol levels.
If you like garlic, there's no reason not to add it to your favourite
dishes.

Benefits of Fish Oil

International studies have found less heart disease in people who
eat fish regularly. It has been shown that Eskimos in Greenland
who eat nearly a pound of fish a day have low rates of death from
heart disease. This may well be due to the health benefits of fish
oils containing omega-3 fatty acids, which help to make the blood
thinner and less likely to clot, help protect the delicate linings of
arteries, and may also lower blood pressure.

Rich dietary sources of omega-3 include cold water fish such as
salmon, trout, mackerel, sardines and herring. Specifically there
are three groups of men who may benefit from fish oil, either in
dietary form or supplements. Firstly, men who already have coronary heart disease are recommended to eat one portion of oily fish
a day. Secondly, for men who suffer from arrhythmias – irregular
heart beats – the omega-3 fatty acids in fish oil can stabilise electrical activity in the heart and calm arrhythmias. Thirdly, men with
high levels of triglycerides (blood fat), can benefit because fish oil
supplements have been shown to help lower triglycerides.

Fibre

Fibre comes in two forms: water soluble and insoluble. It is the soluble fibre that helps reduce cholesterol levels. It does this in two ways. Firstly, high-bulk food fills us up and leaves less room for fat in the diet. Secondly, it helps the body to clear LDL cholesterol from the system, which lowers the level of LDL in the blood. Good sources of soluble fibre include oat bran, beans, peas, lentils and corn. Pectin, a soluble fibre found in such fruits as apples, citrus fruits, cranberries and sour plums, can also reduce high cholesterol levels. Wheat bran, which is an insoluble fibre, has no direct effect on cholesterol.

HDL Cholesterol

Secondly, the good guy: HDL cholesterol, which I call 'happy' cholesterol. High levels of HDL cholesterol can help protect you from heart disease. HDL cholesterol is called good cholesterol because it mops up excess LDL cholesterol left behind in your arteries and carries it to the liver, where it is broken down and passed out of the body. It also helps to impede hardening of the blood vessel walls by preventing LDL from causing damage. There is increasing evidence now that low HDL cholesterol (i.e. a HDL value of less than 1 mmol/litre) is an independent risk factor for heart disease. So, keeping your HDL or happy cholesterol high, in other words keeping it over 1, helps to protect against heart disease. It appears that the higher the HDL the more protection you get.

So Not All Cholesterol Is Bad For Me Then?

Absolutely not. HDL cholesterol is good for your health. Unfortunately many men suffer from low HDL cholesterol. Research has shown that smoking, raised blood pressure, diabetes and being overweight are associated with low HDL cholesterol.

So What Can I Do to Raise My HDL Cholesterol Levels?

There are a number of things you can do to raise your HDL cholesterol levels:

- If you are overweight (have a BMI greater than 25) then weight
  reduction can help boost your HDL levels.
- Regular exercise has shown to be very beneficial for boosting
  HDL cholesterol levels. The key is *regular* exercise. Finding that
  time in the day to squeeze in a 30 to 40 minute walk may be all
  that is required.
- If you smoke, stop!
- The consumption of 1 or 2 units of alcohol daily has been shown
  to elevate the HDL cholesterol levels. At one time the flavinoids
  found in red wine, which are powerful antioxidants, were
  thought to have the most beneficial effect. However, it is now
  thought that any form of alcohol can have this HDL-
  elevating effect. However, it is important to recognise that, at
  levels of more than 1 or 2 units per day, this beneficial effect of
  alcohol on heart disease is reversed and the heart protective benefits are lost. For some people the negative effects of even 1 to 2
  units of alcohol on physical or mental well-being are greater
  than any potential benefits to be gained from raising the HDL
  level.
- A heart-healthy diet, which is high in fish oils and low in starchy
  carbohydrates, is beneficial for HDL cholesterol.
- For dark chocolate lovers, however, chocolate that is rich in cocoa
  is beneficial for HDL cholesterol. Cocoa is a powerful antioxidant, and dark chocolate is rich in cocoa. Look for those types
  with greater than 70–85 per cent cocoa.
- Vitamin B_3, also known as niacin, is very effective at increasing
  HDL cholesterol levels and may do so by up to 30 per cent. This

can be taken in vitamin supplement form or can be prescribed as medication. Flushing of the face and tummy side effects can be a problem with high-dose niacin.

Triglycerides

Triglycerides are a type of fat found in the blood. Too much triglyceride in your blood can increase your chances of heart disease. There are many reasons why your blood fat may be raised, including:

- Being overweight
- Eating a diet rich in saturated fat, i.e. too many fries, etc.
- Not taking enough exercise
- Alcohol – drinking more than the recommended safe limits of alcohol can cause elevation in blood triglyceride levels.
- Genetic factors, i.e. family history

What Can I Do if My Triglyceride Levels Are Too High?

Make sure your diet is heart-healthy (as for low cholesterol) and eat plenty of oily fish, which is rich in omega-3. Keep your weight down, take plenty of exercise and moderate your alcohol intake.

Sometimes several of the above factors may be involved. So if your blood fat level is raised it is time to look at your diet, maybe, as we suggested earlier, by keeping a food diary over a week or so, not only of what you eat but also of your exercise habits and alcohol intake. Maybe some positive changes can be a key step towards improving, not only your blood cholesterol and blood fat levels, but your overall health as well.

How Can I Check My Cholesterol Level?

A blood test provided by your family doctor can analyse your cholesterol numbers for you. Remember to fast for at least 12 hours prior to this test being taken. Raised LDL and low HDL levels are both independent risk factors for heart disease. Therefore, it is important to know your LDL and HDL values as well as your total cholesterol value and blood fat (triglycerides) level. A 'lipid profile' is the name of the blood test to check total cholesterol as well as HDL cholesterol, LDL cholesterol and blood fat (triglyceride) levels.

How Often Should I Have It Tested?

This depends on your family history and your individual circumstances. There are still a lot of men out there who don't know their cholesterol level, so getting it checked is a good start. If it is raised, your doctor will probably recommend regular monitoring of it and assessing its response to a heart-healthy, low-cholesterol diet. If you are on treatment for high cholesterol then it is recommended that you have it checked every six months or so.

Cholesterol-Lowering Foods and Spreads

There are now a range of foods that can help lower your cholesterol. These foods have ingredients called 'plant stanol esters', which reduce the amount of cholesterol in food absorbed from your stomach into your blood after eating. By doing this they can lower the level of cholesterol in your blood. However, these products don't affect the production of LDL cholesterol in the liver, so if you are programmed to make too much cholesterol then you will continue to make too much regardless of what you eat or when.

There are a variety of these food products for sale in supermarkets and they include spreads, yogurts and milk. They may help if your cholesterol level is high but they are no substitute for a heart-healthy diet. Examples on the Irish market include Benecol and Flora Pro.Activ. These products can also be expensive. Talk to your doctor to see if they may be suitable for you.

Cholesterol in Your Genes

Sometimes dietary and lifestyle changes don't result in cholesterol levels returning to normal. This may be because you have a genetic predisposition to make too much cholesterol, in which case, no matter how healthy your diet is, your liver is still going to make too much LDL cholesterol at night. This can cause confusion because it is often wrongly assumed that if your cholesterol is up then it must be your diet that's causing it. Some Irish men are simply genetically programmed to make too much cholesterol – for them it is all in the genes. In my experience, for most men it's a bit of both: a sub-optimal diet and lifestyle, often with a family history of heart disease and a genetic predisposition. A good start is getting your cholesterol checked and then having a discussion with your family doctor about the significance of the results.

Medical Treatments to Lower Your Cholesterol

A family of drugs known as statins, of which there are several types, can be used to lower your cholesterol levels. They work by blocking the production of LDL cholesterol in the liver. This means that the amount of cholesterol that can be dumped into the blood is decreased and, at the same time, the amount of LDL the liver can remove from the blood is increased. The result of this process is lowered total and LDL cholesterol values. Statins are also believed to have an anti-inflammatory benefit on the coronary arteries, so that they tend to stabilise blockages and reduce the risk of potentially life-threatening clots being created.

Many studies have shown the benefits of statins in terms of reducing the risk of heart attack and stroke, which are two common long-term complications of raised LDL cholesterol levels. The bottom line is that the effectiveness of statins is beyond question.

Clinical studies show that these drugs can lower LDL cholesterol by up to 60 per cent and raise HDL cholesterol by up to 10 per cent. Large studies of statins show that the use of these drugs is associated with a 20 to 30 per cent reduction in death and in the incidence of major cardiovascular events, such as heart attacks, strokes and angina.

For most people, statins seem to be fairly well tolerated, with the most commonly described side effects including abdominal wind and sometimes muscle aches. Less common effects include nausea and drowsiness. Hair loss has also been described. These side effects are relatively uncommon. However, serious side effects can occasionally occur and regular monitoring is essential.

Statins are known to cause muscle problems. On rare occasions severe muscle aches and pains can occur, which usually reverse on stopping the drug. A rare but potentially serious side effect is where the muscles break down. This is called rhabdomyolysis and can lead to kidney failure and even death. This is thought to affect about one in every fifty thousand people who take statins. Therefore it is important to be vigilant about side effects and discuss them with your doctor. Statins are broken down through the liver so it is advised that a liver blood test be done at six monthly intervals to check liver function.

At least five statins are currently on the market in Ireland: atorvastatin (Lipitor), fluvastatin (Lescol), pravastatin (Lipostat), rosuvastatin (Crestor) and simvastatin (Zocor).

Studies on the long-term safety of statins are reassuring so far. This is important, as most people prescribed statins will probably need to take these drugs for many years. There does not appear to be any evidence of an increased risk of death from non-cardiac causes.

Ultimately, the decision as to whether you need a statin to treat your cholesterol is best taken in consultation with your family doctor. He or she will be able to advise you of the pros and cons in your particular case.

As doctors, we try to look at your overall risk of heart disease, which takes into account several risk factors including your age, whether or not you smoke, your blood pressure, your blood sugar levels, your weight and your family history. It is almost always better to try out a cholesterol-lowering, heart-healthy diet for several months before embarking on medication. Having said that, there is no doubt that many lives have been saved since statins arrived on the scene.

Key Points

- Many Irish men have raised cholesterol levels. Raised cholesterol is an important risk factor for heart disease and stroke, which are the most common causes of premature death and disability in Irish men.
- High cholesterol is a risk factor you can do something about (just like smoking, blood pressure, excess weight, lack of exercise, poor diet and stress). As the saying goes, have the courage to change the things you can.
- It's important to know your numbers, not just your total cholesterol figure but also your LDL, HDL and blood triglyceride levels.
- A heart-healthy diet is good for your heart health and usually helps lower cholesterol.
- For some men, it's all in the genes; no matter what they eat, their cholesterol levels remain high.
- Cholesterol-lowering medication is very effective and safe for most people with raised cholesterol.
- Knowledge is power. By understanding your risk factors for heart disease, including cholesterol, you are in a better position to make positive changes. Good luck!

7

Cancer – The Big 'C'

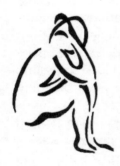

Cancer is a serious health issue for Irish men. About one in every three Irish men will develop cancer at some stage in their lives and about one in six men will die from it. The word 'cancer' is often perceived as a frightening one, yet cancer is not the hopeless diagnosis it once was. Many cancers can now be prevented through the combination of a healthy lifestyle and regular check-ups. Those cancers that can be detected early can be treated before it is too late. Unfortunately, research has shown that Irish men tend to ignore warning symptoms and present late to their doctor for check-ups and medical advice. Through a combination of fear, denial, embarrassment and lack of time, men often ignore their own health, to their cost. The national cancer registry has shown that rates of common cancers in Irish men are set to increase by over 50 per cent by 2020. The four most common cancers in men are:

- Skin cancer
- Prostate cancer (discussed in Chapter 8)

- Colon cancer
- Lung cancer

What Is Cancer?

The basic unit in the body is the cell and we all have billions of cells in our bodies. Normally, cells divide to make more cells when the body needs to either repair existing cells or replace those that have worn out or died. This process of cell growth, repair, death and renewal is normally finely tuned and regulated. It is a continual process and helps to keep our bodies in good shape.

The main feature that all cancers have in common is a lack of regulated or proper cell growth. The inbuilt system of checks and balances breaks down. So when a cancer cell begins to grow, it multiplies out of control. If cells keep dividing when new cells are not needed, a mass of tissue forms. This mass of extra tissue is called a 'growth' or 'tumour'.

Benign and Malignant Tumours

Tumours can be benign or malignant. What's the difference? Benign tumours are not cancer and are rarely a threat to life. Cells from benign tumours do not spread to other parts of the body. They can usually be removed surgically or treated with drugs and/or radiation to reduce their size and, in most cases, they do not recur. Malignant tumours are cancer. There are more than 100 different types. Cancer cells can invade and damage tissues and organs near the tumour as well as spreading to form new malignant tumours in other parts of the body. This spread of cancer is called metastasis (pronounced me-tas-tis-iss). The word cancer itself comes from the Latin word for crab. This is because historically the swollen blood vessels around the area of a tumour were thought to resemble a crab's limbs.

What Causes Cancer?

As we have said, cancer occurs when the fine-tuning mechanism in the body that controls and regulates cell growth and cell death is altered. In addition, the body's natural immune system, which is normally able to kill off many cancer cells, malfunctions. The result of these two events is uncontrolled cell growth and these cells can then invade other parts of the body.

This can occur because of genetic factors or environmental factors or a combination of both. Many people are genetically programmed to develop cancer. In other words, if there is a strong history of cancer in the family then you may be more at risk of developing that type of cancer yourself. Bowel cancer is a good example of this. Environmental factors include exposure to a wide variety of substances that are known to increase the risk of getting cancer. These substances are known as carcinogens.

Known Risk Factors for Cancer

A risk factor is anything that increases a person's chance of getting a disease such as cancer. Different cancers have different risk factors. Several risk factors make a person more likely to develop cancer:

- Cigarette smoking and tobacco use. Smokers worldwide account for about 85 per cent of cases of lung cancer in men. Smoking is also a major cause of oesophageal, mouth, throat, bladder and pancreatic cancer. There are over fifty different carcinogens in tobacco smoke.
- Obesity
- A high-saturated-fat 'Western diet'. Lots of red meat and little fresh fruit and vegetables lead to an increased risk of both colon and prostate cancer.
- Lack of exercise

- Exposure to workplace carcinogens such as asbestos, arsenic, benzene and vinyl chloride
- Drinking large amounts of alcohol leads to an increased risk of mouth, throat, oesophageal and liver cancer.
- Genetic factors are important in some cancers, such as colon, stomach and prostate cancer.
- Exposure to radon gas. This is a natural radioactive gas which seeps from the ground into the home. Levels of radon are quite high in various parts of Ireland and it is strongly associated with lung cancer.
- Food additives such as nitrates in processed foods, which are converted in the body to carcinogenic nitrosamines
- Barbequing food may produce carcinogenic chemicals such as polycyclic aromatic hydrocarbons that may promote intestinal cancer.
- Medical treatment that suppresses the immune system, allowing for successful organ transplantation, can also result in cancer because of this suppression of the immune system.
- Radiation
  - sunlight exposes the body to ultraviolet radiation. Ultraviolet radiation over a prolonged period of time can damage DNA and cause cancer. This is why excess sunbathing or sunburn can cause skin cancer.
  - other forms of ionising radiation such as nuclear energy (think of the Chernobyl tragedy), medical x-rays and the natural gamma radiation in cosmic rays

- Infections
  - virus infections associated with cancer would include the HIV virus, which weakens and destroys the body's natural defence system, thereby opening the door to many cancers.

o hepatitis B and C viruses can lead to liver cancer.
o the human papillomavirus, which is sexually transmitted by men to women, can cause cervical cancer in women.
o *Helicobacter pylori*, a bacterial infection, if untreated is associated with an increased risk of stomach cancer.

<u>Length of Exposure</u>

Of course the likelihood of developing cancer from a carcinogen increases in relation to the intensity and length of exposure to that carcinogen. For example, someone who continues to eat a diet high in saturated animal fat and low in fresh fruit and vegetables is at higher risk of bowel and prostate cancer than a man who may have had a poor diet but has now made some positive changes. Smoking one cigarette once clearly has a negligible risk of lung cancer compared to smoking twenty cigarettes a day for thirty years.

Radon

Radon is the second leading cause of lung cancer after cigarette smoking. The World Health Organization has classified radon as a Class 1 carcinogen. When breathed into the lungs this radioactive gas damages lung tissues, which can lead to lung cancer. Radon is a naturally occurring gas that comes from the radioactive decay of uranium in our rocks and soils. It has no odour, colour or taste and so can not be detected by humans. There are parts of Ireland where radon gas levels are very high, including the south east. Radon dissolves and is harmless in the open air but in enclosed spaces like houses it can build up to dangerous levels. All new houses now have to be fitted with a radon barrier but any house built prior to 1998 does not have to have a radon barrier fitted. Therefore it is important to check radon levels in your own house. This can be done quite simply by getting a radon counter, which is available from the Radiological Protection Institute of Ireland in Dublin (RPII) (www.rpii.ie). The counter is left in your house for a period of time and then sent back to them for analysis. If the radon levels are high, then remedial measures can be taken to correct this. According to the RPII, radon accounts for about two-thirds of the total radiation to which the average Irish person is exposed. The lifetime risk of lung cancer for a 70-year-old man who has been exposed to high levels of radon is one in fifty.

General Warning Signs of Cancer – Catch it Early

While cancer is best prevented, early detection is vital to maximise the chance of cure. This means, as a man, you must be aware of potential early warning signs of cancer and take appropriate action. While many men with some of the listed symptoms won't actually have cancer or other serious illnesses, it's important not to take chances with your health. If in doubt, check it out! There really are no advantages to delaying seeking medical advice. On the contrary, early detection can literally sometimes be the difference between life and death.

- Any change in your bowel habit such as bleeding from the back passage, constipation or diarrhoea, or a feeling of incomplete emptying may indicate early bowel cancer.
- A change in your waterworks pattern, including urinating more often, the stream stopping and starting, peeing at night and with a sense of urgency, may indicate prostate problems.
- A sore that doesn't heal can suggest mouth or skin cancer.
- Any obvious change in a mole or a wart, such as an increase in size, change in colour or bleeding, may indicate skin cancer.
- Unusual bleeding from any site of the body:
  - blood in the stool may indicate colon cancer.
  - blood in the urine may indicate bladder cancer or kidney cancer.
  - spitting or coughing up blood may indicate lung cancer.

- A lump or swelling in the testicles may indicate testicular cancer.
- Persistent heartburn, indigestion, difficulty swallowing or feeling something getting stuck may indicate cancer of the food pipe (oesophagus) or stomach.
- A persistent cough or chronic hoarseness may be a sign of throat or lung cancer.
- Any nagging pain in the bones or elsewhere without apparent reason
- Unexplained weight loss or loss of appetite
- Persistent sweating
- Low-grade fever
- Unexplained bruising
- Persistent headaches
- Unusual fatigue

Treatment Options for Cancer

Surgical removal of the tumour is usually the best treatment option if it is possible. Other options include chemotherapy or radiotherapy, which may be used on their own or in combination. The potential for the use of these treatments depends on many factors, including the type and location of the tumour, as well as whether and where else in the body the tumour has spread to. If radiotherapy or chemotherapy is used to treat a cancer along with surgery then this is called adjuvant chemotherapy or adjuvant radiotherapy.

Chemotherapy is medication that attacks cancer cells. Some forms can be given orally while others are given by injection into the blood vessels. There are different chemotherapy 'cocktails' used for different tumours. One of the main side effects of this treatment is a weakening of the immune system.

Radiotherapy is a treatment that uses beams of radiation to attack cancer cells. This is usually external to the body but recently, for prostate and breast cancers, radiation capsules are sometimes being placed inside the body to irradiate the tumour from the inside out.

Lung Cancer

Lung cancer usually starts in the lining of the tubes that bring air into the lungs. Lung cancers are believed to develop slowly over a period of many years.

What Are the Symptoms of Lung Cancer?

Lung cancer usually does not show symptoms when it first develops, but symptoms often appear when the tumour begins growing. Each individual may experience symptoms differently.

A persistent cough is the most common symptom of lung cancer. Other symptoms include:

- Hoarseness
- Blood-streaked sputum or phlegm (spit)
- Constant chest pain
- Feeling short of breath
- Wheezing
- Recurring lung infections, such as pneumonia or bronchitis
- Unexplained fever
- Low sodium levels, leading to confusion

Like all cancers, lung cancer can cause general symptoms such as loss of energy, fatigue, weight loss, loss of appetite, non-specific aches and pains, headaches and fractures. Direct pressure effects on large blood vessels or certain nerves near the lung can cause swelling of the neck and face or cause pain and weakness in the shoulder, arm or hand. Of course, some or all of these symptoms can be caused by many other conditions so make sure you consult your doctor for advice.

What Are the Main Risk Factors for Lung Cancer?

By far and away the most common cause of lung cancer is cigarette smoke. Heavy smokers are twenty-five times more likely to get lung cancer than non-smokers. The risk of lung cancer also applies to light smokers, who are ten times more likely to get lung cancer than non-smokers. Passive smoking, in other words breathing in someone else's smoke, is also an increased risk factor for lung cancer.

Rarer causes of lung cancer include exposure to environmental carcinogens such as asbestos, arsenic or radon gas. The effects of exposure to these carcinogens can be much more lethal in smokers.

Smoking marijuana can result in even more tar getting to the lungs than cigarettes and is a recognised cause of lung cancer. As marijuana is an illegal substance, it is not possible to control whether it contains other harmful substances such as pesticides or other additives. Marijuana joints tend to be inhaled very deeply and smoked all the way to the end, where the tar content is the highest.

Chronic inflammation of the lungs such as from tuberculosis, some types of pneumonia and air pollution can also be potential risk factors for lung cancer.

Prevention of Lung Cancer

Lung cancer kills more men than any other cancer worldwide. The vast majority of all lung cancer cases in men are related to smoking. Avoid cigarette smoke, including second-hand smoke. If you smoke cigarettes, stop.

Avoid exposure to environmental pollutants such as asbestos, arsenic, radon and air pollution. Eat well; a diet rich in natural antioxidants such as plenty of fresh fruit and vegetables may have some protective benefits. Make sure you get at least five portions of fresh fruit and vegetables a day. Keep your alcohol consumption within safe limits.

How Is Lung Cancer Diagnosed?

In addition to a complete medical history and a physical examination, procedures used to diagnose lung cancer may include the following:

- A chest x-ray – to look for any mass or spot on the lungs
- Bronchoscopy – this is where a thin flexible tube with a good light source is put into the main tubes of the lungs. This test helps to evaluate and diagnose lung problems, assess blockages and obtain samples of tissue and/or fluid.
- A CAT scan is sometimes used; this can show detailed images of any part of the body and is much more detailed than an x-ray.
- Sputum cytology – the study of phlegm (spit) cells under a microscope.
- Needle biopsy – this is where a sample of the mass is removed and evaluated under a microscope. This can help determine which type of lung cancer you have.
- Other types of scan such as MRI scans, bone scans or PET scans may be needed to determine if the cancer has spread from where it started into other areas of the body.

Treatment for Lung Cancer

Surgery, radiation therapy and chemotherapy may all be used in the treatment of lung cancer. Surgical removal is the treatment of choice if this is possible. Sometimes this can be done successfully. However, if there are multiple tumours or if the tumour is too close to the big blood vessels in the lungs, then non-surgical options need to be considered, including radiotherapy and/or chemotherapy. Some types of lung cancer are more susceptible to chemotherapy than others. This is a decision that your cancer specialist will help you with, taking account not only of your individual medical history, but also your own preferences and wishes.

Colon Cancer

Colon cancer (also known as bowel cancer or colorectal cancer) is the second most common cancer in Irish men. About 1,800 cases are diagnosed in Ireland each year and the average lifetime risk for men is about 3 per cent. Colon cancer is both preventable and curable. It can be prevented by removing pre-cancerous colon polyps (see below). It can be cured if it is found early and surgically removed before it spreads to other parts of the body. However, colon cancer remains a major cause of death and disease in Irish men. The rates of colon cancer are predicted to increase by 50 per cent by the year 2020. Early detection of colon cancer can improve the chances of a cure and overall survival.

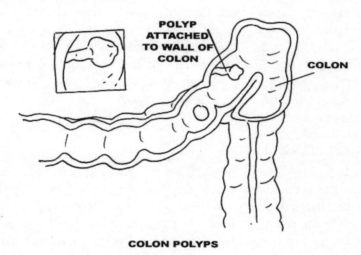

POLYP ATTACHED TO WALL OF COLON

COLON

COLON POLYPS

What Is the Colon?

The colon is a long, muscular hollow tube about 6 feet long and is the part of the digestive system where waste material is stored. It receives undigested food from the small intestine. It removes water from the undigested food, stores it and then finally eliminates it from the body through bowel movements. The rectum is the end of the colon beside the anus or back passage.

What Are the Risk Factors for Colon Cancer?

Factors that have been shown to increase a man's risk of colon cancer include a diet high in fat, polyps in the colon, a family history of colorectal cancer and medical conditions such as ulcerative colitis.

Diet and Colon Cancer

Diets high in saturated fat are believed to increase the risks of colon cancer. In countries with high rates of bowel cancer, the fat intake by the population is much higher than in countries with low cancer rates. Breakdown products of fat metabolism are thought to lead to the formation of cancer-causing chemicals (carcinogens). Diets high in vegetables and high-fibre foods such as wholegrain breads and cereals may rid the bowel of these carcinogens and help reduce the risk of cancer.

Colon Polyps and Colon Cancer

Polyp is the name given to small mushroom-like growths that can appear on the lining of the colon. Colon polyps are initially benign but over years can acquire additional chromosome damage to become cancerous. Some polyps can be pre-cancerous but can be present for many years before they turn into cancer. Doctors believe that most colon cancers develop in colon polyps. Therefore, removing benign colon polyps can prevent colorectal cancer. This can be easily done during a colonoscopy (see pages 121–122).

Know Your Genes – The Genetics of Colon Cancer

Your genetic makeup is an important colon cancer risk factor. The lifetime risk of developing colon cancer is thought to be about 3 per cent. But, if a first degree relative (parent, sibling or child) has bowel cancer then your lifetime risk increases to 9 per cent. However, despite this hereditary risk, most colon cancers still occur in patients who have no family history of colon cancer.

Men who have hereditary colon cancer syndrome tend to develop large numbers of colon polyps at a young age, and are at a very high risk of developing colon cancer early in life. Such a person can develop hundreds or thousands of colon polyps, starting during the teenage years, and is almost certain to develop colon cancer from these polyps by the age of 40. They are also at risk of developing cancers in other organs. Treatment involves removal of the colon at an early age.

Other men start to develop many colonic polyps, which eventually become cancerous, from the age of 30 onwards. Hence it is important to know your family history and get yourself properly checked out.

Ulcerative Colitis and Colon Cancer

Chronic ulcerative colitis is a condition that causes inflammation of the lining of the colon. Colon cancer is a recognised complication of chronic ulcerative colitis and is related to the location and the extent of the disease. Therefore, if you suffer from this condition, regular colonoscopies are recommended to look for pre-cancerous changes.

Other Risk Factors for Colon Cancer

Cigarette smoking has been associated with an increased risk of colon cancer. Patients with diabetes are more likely to be diagnosed with colon cancer. Obesity is associated with an increased risk, as is having a beer belly. Excess alcohol (more than 4 units per day), particularly beer consumption, is an associated risk factor for colon cancer.

What Are the Symptoms of Colon Cancer?

Bowel symptoms may include some or all of the following:

- A persistent change in bowel habit, such as constipation, diarrhoea or alternating constipation and diarrhoea
- Bleeding from the back passage
- Narrow stools
- A feeling of incomplete emptying of the bowel when going to the toilet
- A straining feeling or discomfort in the back passage
- Abdominal pain, cramps or bloating

Colon cancer can be present for several years before symptoms develop. Other symptoms of colon cancer can include fatigue, nausea, weakness, loss of appetite and weight loss. Symptoms vary according to where in the large bowel the tumour is located. The right side of the colon is spacious, and cancers in this area can get big before they cause any abdominal symptoms. These cancers tend to cause iron deficiency anaemia due to the slow loss of blood over a long period of time. Iron deficiency anaemia causes fatigue, weakness and shortness of breath.

The left side of the colon is narrower than the right side and cancers here are more likely to cause partial or complete bowel blockage or obstruction. Cancers causing partial bowel obstruction can cause symptoms of constipation, narrowed stools, diarrhoea, abdominal pains, cramps and bloating. Bright red blood in the stool may also indicate a growth near the end of the left side of the colon or rectum.

If you have these symptoms you should see your doctor without delay. However, other conditions, such as irritable bowel syndrome (spastic colon), ulcerative colitis, Crohn's disease, diverticulosis, and peptic ulcer disease, can all have symptoms that mimic colon cancer.

Early diagnosis of bowel cancer is very important because the percentage chance of cure is directly related to how far advanced the condition is when it is diagnosed. So, if bowel cancer is still located within the bowel wall, the chances of cure may be as high as 100 per cent. Tragically, many Irish men fail to report early warning symptoms of bowel cancer and may put up with these symptoms for many months before seeking help. Delay of this sort can spell disaster.

What Tests Can Be Done to Detect Colon Cancer?

There are a number of tests available to detect colon cancer. These include colonoscopies, enemas, blood tests, digital rectal examination and stool occult blood testing, and genetic testing. The diagnosis is confirmed by the pathological analysis of a sample of the colon. Other tests, including scans, are used if the cancer has spread to other parts of the body, particularly the liver or bones.

Colonoscopy

The best test is usually a colonoscopy. This is where a long, thin, flexible tube, about the thickness of a finger, is put into the back passage. It has a camera at one end and a good light source that allows the bowel lining to be thoroughly examined. Any suspicious areas or growths such as polyps can be biopsied (removed) and sent for further analysis.

Screening Colonoscopy

Regular screening reduces the risk of dying from colon cancer. A screening colonoscopy test is recommended for Irish men at average risk generally every few years from the age of 50 upwards. Men with a higher risk of developing colon cancer may need to start this at an earlier age. This includes men who have a first degree relative with either colon cancer or polyps. These men may need to start screening colonoscopies from the age of 40 or sometimes earlier. Therefore it is important to be aware of your family history, as a family history of colon polyps or colon cancer merits close attention to your colon.

Barium Enema

Sometimes an alternative test called a barium enema is done. This involves putting a white, chalky liquid containing barium into the back passage and taking x-ray pictures of the colon afterwards. Tumours and other abnormalities can appear as dark shadows on the x-rays.

Blood Tests

Blood tests can help in the diagnosis. For example, low iron (anaemia) in someone with suspicious symptoms (described above) will point in the direction of further tests. Sometimes, the doctor may obtain a blood test for carcinoembryonic antigen (CEA). CEA is a substance produced by some cancer cells. It is sometimes found in high levels in patients with colon cancer, especially when the disease has spread.

Digital Rectal Examination and Stool Occult Blood Testing

As part of an annual check-up with your own doctor, a digital rectal examination to check your prostate can at the same time examine the lower rectum and detect any low-lying rectal tumours. This is done by inserting a gloved and lubricated index finger into the back passage area. This can be followed by an FOB (faecal occult blood) test, whereby a sample of faeces is sent away to a laboratory to be analysed for the presence of tiny speckles of blood. This can be an important screening test for colon cancers and polyps. Tumours of the colon and rectum tend to bleed slowly into the faeces and the small amount of blood mixed into the faeces is usually not visible to the naked eye. A small amount of faecal sample is smeared on a special card for occult blood testing. Usually three consecutive faecal cards are collected. However, be aware many other conditions can cause occult blood in the faeces. It is also important to realise that if your faeces samples have tested negative for occult blood this does not necessarily mean the absence of colon cancer. Having said that, a man who tests positive for faecal occult blood is thought to have at least a 30 per cent chance of having a colon polyp and a 3 per cent chance of having colon cancer.

Genetic Counselling and Testing

Blood tests are now available to test for hereditary colon cancer syndrome. Families with many cases of colon cancer, especially at a young age, can be referred for genetic counselling followed possibly by genetic testing. The advantages of this process include identifying family members with a high risk of developing colon cancer so as to begin colonoscopies early, as well as alleviating concern for members who test negative for the defect.

Treatment of Colon Cancer

Surgical removal of the affected part of the colon is usually the treatment of choice. After the operation, a colostomy bag would be attached to the skin surface of the stomach wall to collect the faeces.

This can be temporary or permanent, depending on where the cancer is located. Treatment often also requires chemotherapy or radiotherapy, depending on the type of tumour and where it has spread to. Sometimes chemotherapy is done even before surgery to reduce the size of the tumour. The long-term prognosis is related to how far the cancer has spread before it is diagnosed, with men having tumours confined within the wall of the colon doing best.

How Can Bowel Cancer Be Prevented?

The best way to prevent bowel cancer is to eat a diet rich in fibre and fresh fruit and vegetables and low in animal fat. This means less red meat, less processed or cured meats such as bacon, sausages and ham, less fatty processed foods such as cakes, biscuits and chocolate, and less alcohol.

Fibre is the insoluble, non-digestible part of plant material present in fruits, vegetables and wholegrain breads and cereals. It is thought that lots of fibre in your diet leads to the creation of bulky stools that can rid the intestines of potential carcinogens. In addition, fibre speeds up the passage of faecal material through the colon, which allows less time for a potential carcinogen to react with the colon lining.

Apart from a healthy diet and lifestyle, the most effective way to prevent colon cancer is early detection and removal of pre-cancerous colon polyps. Of course, even in cases where cancer has already developed, early detection still significantly improves the chances of a cure by surgically removing the cancer before the disease spreads to other organs.

Regular physical exercise appears to be beneficial in terms of reducing the risk of colorectal cancer. Statins, which are used to treat high cholesterol, have recently been shown to possibly have a protective effect against bowel cancer. Taking supplements of folic acid may have some protective effect on colon cancer. Other agents being evaluated as possibly helping to prevent colon cancer include calcium, selenium and Vitamins A, C and E. More studies are needed before these agents can be recommended for widespread use by the public to prevent colon cancer. Taking low-dose aspirin can also have some protective benefit against bowel cancer. However, the flip side of this is that regular aspirin can slightly increase your risk of bleeding. Discuss the potential benefits of low-dose aspirin with your family doctor.

Unfortunately, colon cancers can be well advanced before they are detected. Being aware of the early warning signs of bowel cancer is important, so you can seek immediate help if need be.

Stomach Cancer

Stomach cancer remains one of the most common forms of cancer. However, the worldwide incidence of stomach cancer has declined rapidly over recent decades. Part of the decline may be due to awareness and treatment of helicobacter infection (see below). The increased use of refrigerators in recent decades has improved the storage of food and means that fresh food and vegetables (a valuable source of antioxidants important for cancer prevention) are more easily available. It has also led to a reduction in bacterial and fungal contamination, as well as salt-based preservation of food.

Symptoms to suggest stomach cancer include vague discomfort in the abdomen, loss of appetite, indigestion, heartburn or ulcer-like symptoms, a sense of fullness after eating a small meal, nausea, vomiting and abdominal swelling. Unfortunately, stomach cancer usually has no symptoms until the later stages. The optimal treatment of stomach cancer is the subject of ongoing research and usually involves some combination of surgery, chemotherapy and radiotherapy.

Causes of Stomach Cancer

The exact cause of stomach cancer is unknown. However, cigarette smoking and alcohol abuse increase the risk of stomach cancer. Dietary factors implicated in stomach cancer include a high-salt, processed-food diet with little fresh fruit and vegetables. Processed foods often contain nitrates, which can then be converted in the body to nitrosamines – potentially potent carcinogens. Stomach cancer is twice as common in men as in women. Infection of the stomach with the bacteria *Helicobacter pylori* is an important risk factor for stomach cancer.

Prevention of Stomach Cancer

As well as general advice regarding not smoking and not abusing alcohol, it is important to eat a good diet: one rich in fresh fruit, vegetables and beans, and with plenty of wholegrain breads and pasta. Processed foods and smoked foods should be avoided. As a man you should consider getting yourself tested for the presence of *Helicobacter pylori*.

What Is Helicobacter Pylori (H. Pylori)?

H. pylori is a spiral-shaped bacterium found in the stomach, which (along with acid secretion) can damage the stomach and part of the bowel known as the duodenum. It is the leading cause of ulcers. It was discovered by an Australian medical student in 1991 – quite a breakthrough as up until then nothing was thought to be able to live in the strongly acidic environment of the stomach. It is not known what causes certain people to develop *H. pylori*. In recent years it has been shown to be a risk factor for stomach cancer and is now classified as a carcinogen. Therefore it is worth getting tested for it and treated. Most people will never have symptoms or problems related to *H. pylori* infection. When symptoms are present, they may include a multitude of stomach-related symptoms, including heartburn, bloating and wind, as well as tummy discomfort, which may be relieved by eating. Always consult your doctor to have your symptoms evaluated.

The presence of *Helicobacter pylori* can be diagnosed either by a blood test or by having a gastroscopy, in which a thin flexible tube with a light source is inserted into the stomach to view its inner lining. A sample of tissue can be removed and an on-the-spot test, known as the urease test, can be done to diagnose the presence of *Helicobacter*. Urease is an enzyme made by the *H. pylori* bug. Another option is the hydrogen breath test where you blow into a hydrogen-based machine. *H. pylori* can be successfully treated and eradicated in most cases with a short course of antibiotics combined with a tablet to turn off the acid tap in the stomach. These tests can also be done to ensure proof of cure after treatment to make sure the bug is gone.

Skin Cancer

Skin cancer is a common cancer in Irish men and is on the increase. Unlike many other types of cancer however, only a small minority of those affected by skin cancer will actually die of the condition.

What Are the Different Types of Skin Cancer?

There are three main types of skin cancer. The most common types of skin cancers are basal cell (BCC) and squamous cell (SCC) skin cancers. These can be disfiguring but are unlikely to spread to other parts of the body and so are rarely fatal. The least common form of skin cancer is also the most dangerous and is called malignant melanoma.

Basal Cell Cancer

This is the most common type of skin cancer and accounts for about 75 per cent of all cases. It often looks like a small, raised pearl-like bump or nodule on a sun-exposed area of skin on the head, face, neck or back of the hands. It can easily be mistaken for a sore that doesn't heal. This highly treatable cancer tends to start in the top layer of skin and grows very slowly. It commonly occurs among persons with light-coloured eyes, hair and complexion. Untreated, it can eventually spread down through the skin, which is why it has the alternative medical term of a 'rodent ulcer'.

Squamous Cell Cancer

This is the second most common form of skin cancer and accounts for about 20 per cent of cases. It often looks like a raised crusted lesion on the sun-exposed areas of skin. Symptoms may include any spot or sore on the skin that changes or fails to heal, as well as localised scaliness, oozing, bleeding, itching, tenderness or pain at the site of the spot. Squamous cell carcinoma, although more aggressive than basal cell carcinoma, is highly treatable. It may appear as nodules or red, scaly patches of skin, and may be found on the face, ears, lips and mouth. Squamous cell carcinoma, if untreated, can spread to other parts of the body. This type of skin cancer is usually found in fair-skinned people.

Malignant Melanoma

Malignant melanoma is the least common but most dangerous form of skin cancer. It affects about 500 people each year in Ireland and its incidence is on the rise. Risk factors for developing malignant melanoma include a history of melanoma in the family. Those with certain skin types are at increased risk of melanoma, particularly those who are fair-skinned with blue eyes, and men who develop lobster-type skin after a few days in the sun. Having a lot of moles on your skin is termed dysplastic naevus syndrome and is associated with an increased lifetime risk of developing melanoma. Some people are born with very large moles on their bodies that are at increased risk of turning into melanoma over the long term.

Malignant melanoma starts in the melanocyte cells that produce pigment in the skin. It usually begins as a mole that then turns cancerous. This cancer may spread quickly.

Diagnosis

The warning signs for melanoma are either the arrival of a new mole or a change in an existing mole. The most useful signs in a mole are:

- An increase in size
- A change in shape
- A change in colour
- Bleeding, crusting, itching or altered sensation

Also look out for the ABCD of mole changes, which are a red alert for possible melanoma:

- **A**symmetry – one half of the mole different from the other
- **B**order – an irregular edge to the mole
- **C**olour – colour variation within the mole, i.e. light and dark brown areas
- **D**iameter – generally moles greater than 6 millimetres in diameter (the end of a pencil)

Any new or existing mole with these changes must be fully removed. As with many other cancers, early detection greatly increases the chance of long-term cure as the survival rate from melanoma is directly related to the depth and thickness of the mole at the time of removal. If you are concerned or unsure about any mark or mole on your skin, discuss this with your family doctor.

What Are the Risk Factors for Skin Cancer?

- Skin cancer is more common in fair-skinned people, especially those with blond or red hair and those who have light-coloured eyes.
- A family history of melanoma.
- Sun exposure – the main risk factor is ultraviolet light and sunburn. In particular, blistering sunburns in childhood and adolescence significantly increase the risk of developing malignant melanoma. Overexposure to ultraviolet radiation from the sun can cause skin cancer. Sun exposure between 10 a.m. and 4 p.m. is most intense and therefore most harmful.
- Sunbed use is associated with skin cancer, including melanoma.
- Many ordinary moles on the skin (more than fifty).
- Funny-shaped moles (known as dysplastic naevi).
- Chronic non-healing wounds, especially burns.
- Those who work outdoors, such as construction workers and farmers, have increased risk.

Know Your Skin, Know Your Moles

It is important to examine your skin on a regular basis and become familiar with moles, freckles and other skin blemishes. This will allow you to better identify changes at an early stage. Be alert to changes in the number, size, shape and colour of pigmented areas. Finding suspicious moles or skin cancer early is the key to treating skin cancer successfully. Some moles are not easy to watch, particularly those on the back, so you may need your partner's help here. Getting your moles looked at as part of a check-up with your doctor is also a good idea. Sometimes taking a photo of a mole allows you to see if it is changing over time.

Treatment of Skin Cancer

Most skin cancers are treated by simply removing the lesion. This is then analysed in the pathology laboratory under the microscope to confirm the diagnosis. Sometimes small non-melanoma skin cancers can be successfully treated by freezing the cancer off or by radiation treatment.

For melanoma, subsequent treatment will depend on how far the condition has spread prior to diagnosis. Interferon, a drug that alters the immune system, is sometimes used to treat patients with melanoma.

Prevention of Skin Cancer

The best way to prevent skin cancer is to be sun aware and protect your skin:

- Avoid sunburn and avoid excessive sun exposure. Minimise exposure to the midday sun (10 a.m. to 4 p.m.), when the sun is highest in the sky.
- Apply sunscreen all over your body and regularly use a broad-spectrum sunscreen with an SPF of 15 or higher, even on cloudy days, on all areas of your body that are exposed to the sun. This protects against both UVA and UVB rays.
- Reapply sunscreen every 2 hours, even on cloudy days. Reapply after swimming or perspiring.
- Avoid exposure to UV radiation from sunlamps or tanning parlours.
- Wear protective clothing. Hats should provide shade for both the face and back of the neck. Wearing sunglasses will reduce the

amount of rays reaching the eye by filtering most of the rays. This helps to protect the eyelids as well as the lens.

- Remember, sand and pavements reflect UV rays even under an umbrella. Snow is a particularly good reflector of UV rays. Reflective surfaces can reflect up to 85 per cent of the damaging sun rays. Don't forget your sunscreen on your skiing holiday.

Testicular Cancer

Testicular cancer is a young man's disease. It is the most common form of cancer in men between the ages of 15 and 34. Testicular cancer is the exception to the rule that most cancer occurs in middle-aged or older men. It is more common in white men, for reasons that are unknown.

The incidence of testicular cancer has been increasing in recent years. However it is one of the most curable forms of cancer, provided it is diagnosed early, which is why awareness of it is so important. Practising regular testicular self-examination (see Chapter 12) allows testicular problems, including testicular cancer, to be diagnosed early and cured. Tragically, many men still remain unaware of the importance of this simple and potentially life-saving measure. And many men who are aware still delay unnecessarily before seeking medical help.

Testicular cancer is a 'germ cell cancer' as the cells which become cancerous are those involved with making sperm. Testicular cancers are divided into two main types, depending on the type of cell causing the cancer: seminomas, which occur in about half of all cases, and non-seminomas, which make up the rest and are mainly teratomas, but include some other rare types. It is important to know which kind of cell the cancer started from because these types of cancer may be treated differently.

Symptoms of Testicular Cancer

The following are the most common symptoms of testicular cancer. However, each individual may experience symptoms differently. The symptoms of testicular cancer may resemble other conditions or medical problems. The most common symptoms include:

- A lump in either testicle, usually painless
- Enlargement of a testicle
- A feeling of heaviness in the scrotum
- A dull ache in the lower abdomen or groin
- A sudden collection of fluid in the scrotum
- Pain or discomfort in a testicle or the scrotum
- Enlargement or tenderness of the breasts

What Causes Testicular Cancer?

The exact cause of testicular cancer is not known. In many cases testicular cancer develops for no apparent reason. However, there are a number of risk factors that can increase the risk of getting the disease:

- Age – most testicular cancers occur in young men between the ages of 15 and 40.
- A history of an undescended testicle(s). This increases the risk of testicular cancer in later life, which is why an undescended testis should always be 'brought down' into the scrotum. This allows any later changes in it to be detected at an early stage.
- Family history of testicular cancer
- A personal history of cancer in the other testicle
- Race/ethnicity – the rate of testicular cancer is higher in white men than in other population groups, which suggests that some genetic or environmental factor is involved.
- HIV infection

- Men whose mothers took a hormone called DES (diethylstilbe-strol) during pregnancy to prevent miscarriage.

Can Testicular Cancer Be Prevented?

Currently, we don't know if or how testicular cancer can be prevented because there is no known cause of the disease; many of the suggested risk factors are those that cannot be changed and many men who get testicular cancer do not have the suggested risk factors.

How Is Testicular Cancer Diagnosed?

The key is to notice any lump or abnormality in the testes and get this checked out by your doctor. However, it is important to remember that most lumps or abnormalities detected are not cancer. If you are suspicious about a testicular swelling then further tests may include the following:

- Ultrasound – a simple and painless diagnostic scan where gel is put on the scrotum and a probe is used to look at the testes. This test can help tell if the lump is likely to be a tumour or a benign fluid-filled cyst.
- Blood tests – certain blood proteins, known as tumour markers, can be raised in men with testicular cancer. Blood tests that measure these tumour markers can be used to help confirm the diagnosis and also as a means of monitoring treatment.
- Biopsy – a procedure in which a sample of testicular tissue is removed with a needle or during surgery for detailed analysis to determine if cancer or other abnormal cells are present.

If you are confirmed to have testicular cancer then further tests, including scans, are carried out to see if it has spread elsewhere in the body. This helps to determine the best treatment plan.

Treatment for Testicular Cancer

There are several kinds of treatment for testicular cancer. The treatment advised for each case depends on various factors, such as the type of cancer (seminoma or non-seminoma), how far it has spread and your general health.

Surgical removal of the affected testicle is advised in almost all cases. This alone may be curative if the cancer is at an early stage and has not spread. Radiotherapy, to destroy cancer cells or slow the rate of growth, may be done after surgery for men with seminoma tumours to prevent recurrence. Chemotherapy using anti-cancer drugs to destroy cancer cells throughout the body has greatly improved the cure rates of both seminomas and non-seminoma testicular tumours.

What Is the Prognosis?

The prognosis is usually good. Most testicular cancers are diagnosed at an early stage, and after treatment over 90 per cent of men are completely cured. Even if the testicular cancer has spread to other parts of the body there is still a good chance of being cured. After treatment you will be monitored regularly for a number of years to make sure the cancer hasn't come back. This will involve blood tests to measure the tumour markers and sometimes scans as well.

If you have one testis removed, it should not affect your sex life. You should still have normal erections and produce sperm and hormones from the other testis, and so can still father children. However, if you have chemotherapy or radiotherapy, this may affect fertility. You should discuss this with your specialist.

Bladder Cancer

The bladder is a triangular-shaped, hollow organ located in the lower abdomen. The role of the bladder is to store urine; its walls relax and expand to store urine, and contract and flatten to empty urine through the urethra. Bladder cancer occurs when there are abnormal, cancerous cells growing in the bladder. Bladder cancer affects men two to three times more frequently than women.

What Are the Risk Factors for Bladder Cancer?

While the exact causes of bladder cancer are not known, there are well-established risk factors, which include the following:

Cigarette Smoking

By far and away the most important cause of bladder cancer is cigarette smoke. Smoking causes about half of the deaths from bladder cancer among men. There are over fifty different carcinogens in tobacco smoke. When these are inhaled through the lungs into the bloodstream these carcinogens eventually end up in the bladder before being excreted through the urine. The disease occurs in smokers twice as often as non-smokers.

Occupational Exposure

Certain occupations and work environments that expose workers to dyes and some organic chemicals appear to increase the risk of developing bladder cancer. Workers in the rubber, chemical, leather, textile, metal and printing industries are exposed to substances such as aniline dye and aromatic amines that may increase their risk of bladder cancer. Other at-risk occupations include hairdressers, machinists, painters and truck drivers.

Chronic Bladder Irritation

Chronic bladder infections or bladder stones may be linked to certain types of bladder cancer. Infection with certain parasites found in tropical regions of the world can increase the risk of bladder cancer.

Other Risk Factors

The risk of developing bladder cancer increases as a man gets older. It is more common in white men and those with a family history of bladder cancer.

What Are the Symptoms of Bladder Cancer?

Every man may experience symptoms differently and, in the early stages, bladder cancer can be asymptomatic. Symptoms may include blood in the urine; this may be visible to the naked eye, in that the urine looks discoloured, or it may be picked up on examination of the urine by your doctor. Other symptoms include pain or discomfort on urination, frequently feeling the urgent need to urinate, frequent urination and pelvic or flank pain. These symptoms of bladder cancer may resemble other medical conditions or problems and it is important to consult your doctor for advice.

How Is Bladder Cancer Diagnosed?

In addition to a complete medical history and physical examination, diagnostic procedures for bladder cancer may include the following:

Laboratory Tests

Tests can be carried out on the urine to check for the presence of blood, chemicals and bacteria. The urine may be examined microscopically or grown in culture to check for infection. Cancerous cells may be detected using the microscope. Blood tests can also be carried out.

Cystoscopy

This is an examination in which a thin flexible tube and viewing device is inserted through the urethra to examine the bladder and urinary tract for structural abnormalities or obstructions, such as tumours or stones. Samples of the bladder tissue (a biopsy) may be removed through the cystoscope for examination under a microscope in the laboratory.

Intravenous Pyelogram (IVP)

This is a series of x-rays of the kidney, ureters and bladder performed after the injection of a contrast dye into the veins. This test is used to detect tumours, abnormalities, kidney stones or any obstructions, and to assess renal blood flow. It may also be used to rule out other diseases or check for spread (metastasis) of the bladder cancer to other areas of the urinary tract.

What Is the Treatment for Bladder Cancer?

About 70–80 per cent of individuals with bladder cancer have superficial and non-invasive tumours. Treatment of these tumours is often very effective and results in an excellent prognosis. Less often, bladder tumours become more invasive and can spread to other organs. Depending on the extent, bladder cancers may be managed with a single therapy or a combination of treatments, including surgery, radiation therapy and chemotherapy.

How Do You Prevent Bladder Cancer?

While there is no known way to prevent bladder cancer, you can reduce your chances of developing the disease. The best way to do this is to quit smoking and avoid any potential exposure to known bladder carcinogens, such as benzene. As with the prevention of other cancers, it is thought that a diet rich in fresh fruit and vegetables and low in saturated fat is helpful. Drinking plenty of fluids and keeping your urine clear at all times allows toxins to be cleared from the body. Drinking lots of fluids may also limit the time that cancer-causing substances present in urine will remain in contact with bladder cells.

Breast Cancer in Men

Breast cancer in men is uncommon. Less than 1 per cent of all breast cancers occur in men. Although men of all ages can be affected with the disease, the average age at diagnosis is between 60 and 70.

What Are the Risk Factors for Breast Cancer in Men?

Risk factors may include a family history of breast cancer in female relatives. Other factors may include radiation exposure and medical conditions associated with high oestrogen states, such as cirrhosis of the liver.

What Are the Symptoms of Breast Cancer in Men and How Is it Treated?

Every man may experience symptoms differently. Symptoms may include breast lumps, nipple inversion, a nipple discharge (sometimes bloody) or atypical pain or a pulling sensation in the breast. Keep in mind that these symptoms of breast cancer may resemble many other medical conditions. It is important to consult your doctor for advice. Overall survival rates are similar to that of women with breast cancer.

The main treatment is surgical removal, and other treatment options include radiation therapy and chemotherapy.

Liver Cancer

Liver cancer is a rare cancer in men and usually involves a cancer elsewhere in the body spreading to the liver. The main cause of cancer originating in the liver itself is the hepatitis B virus infection, which is why vaccination against hepatitis B is so important for individuals at risk of contracting it. This virus spreads through contact with infected blood. Other infections that can cause liver cancer include hepatitis C, which is also spread via infected blood and other body fluids. Cirrhosis, usually but not always caused by excess alcohol, can also cause liver cancer. Some foodstuffs such as aflatoxin mould on peanuts, for example, can cause liver cancer.

Symptoms of Liver Cancer

Symptoms of liver cancer include yellow jaundice, loss of appetite, weight loss and pain or swelling in the upper abdomen.

Prevention of Liver Cancer

The best way to prevent liver cancer is to avoid hepatitis B or C infection. The most common form of hepatitis (hepatitis A) is not a risk factor for liver cancer. Hepatitis B and C are spread by contact with contaminated body fluids, most commonly blood or saliva. Practising safe sex, including the use of condoms, and avoiding sharing needles are important. There is a vaccine available to prevent hepatitis B. Unfortunately there is no vaccine available yet for the hepatitis C infection. You can also help prevent liver cancer by avoiding drinking excess alcohol, thereby preventing liver cirrhosis.

Treatment of Liver Cancer

Specific treatment for cancer will be determined by your doctors in consultation with you. Factors to be taken into consideration will include:

- The extent of the cancer – how far it has spread
- Your overall health, age and other medical conditions
- Your tolerance for specific medications, procedures or therapies

- Your ideas, concerns and expectations
- Your opinions or preferences

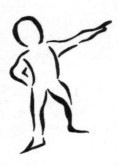

Key Points

- Cancer is common among Irish men. The 'big four' cancers in Irish men are skin, prostate, colon and lung cancers. Testicular cancer is the most common cancer in young men.
- The number of new cancer cases in Irish men may double between 2000 and 2020. Many cancers can be prevented by leading a healthy lifestyle and by being aware of potential warning symptoms and signs. Knowledge is power!

- The good news is that cancer survival is improved by earlier detection and improved treatment.
- Know the ABC of cancer in men:

  - o **A**wareness of the symptoms
  - o **B**e alert to the causes – maximise your chances of preventing cancer
  - o **C**atch it in time – maximise the chance of cure

8

The Prostate

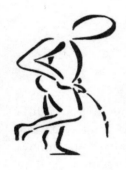

This is definitely one of those male-only health issues, if only for one reason — women don't have one. Yes, boys, we're on our own on this one.

What Is the Prostate?

The prostate is a small male sex gland, about the size and shape of a walnut. However, for such a small gland it packs one hell of a punch. This is because of where it is located in the body. The prostate is found at the bottom of the bladder between the bladder and the penis. It is wrapped around the waterworks tube (known as the urethra).

What Does It Do?

The prostate gland plays an important role in both urinary function and sexual function. The prostate is part of the male reproductive apparatus. It plays a supporting role during sex by producing fluid

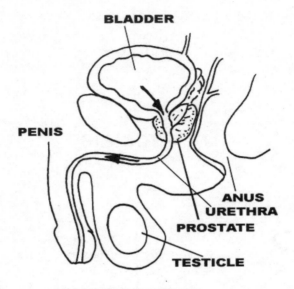

NORMAL PROSTATE

that mixes with sperm at the time of ejaculation. This fluid accounts for most of the milky semen you ejaculate every time you experience an orgasm. This prostate fluid is thought to help nourish sperm and help them reach their target. Prostate fluid also contains a protein known as prostate specific antigen or PSA. The role of PSA is to help liquefy semen, aiding the fertility process. However, some PSA also escapes into the bloodstream. This is the basis of the PSA blood test. It can be a marker of prostate health in that raised levels of PSA in the blood can indicate prostate problems.

The Waterworks System

Understanding the process of urination can help you to understand diseases of the prostate and how they can affect us. When men attempt to urinate, urine passes from the bladder and out of the body through the urethra, a tube that runs from the bladder through the prostate and the penis. The prostate completely surrounds the first part of the urethra. Changes in the prostate, including an increase in size, can put pressure on the urethra, which can then cause symptoms such as needing to urinate more often, difficulty starting to pee, poor stream and dribbling at the end. These are known as 'prostatic symptoms'.

Disorders of the Prostate

There are three main types of prostate disorders:

- Prostatitis
- Benign enlargement of the prostate gland (known as BPH)
- Prostate cancer

Prostatitis

Prostatitis is one of several benign (non-cancerous) conditions causing inflammation of the prostate gland. The prostate is prone to become inflamed and sometimes infected, as it is connected to the processes of both sex and urination. Prostatitis is common and there are estimates that at least half of all men, at some point in their lives, will develop symptoms of this condition. It is not contagious and is not considered to be a sexually transmitted disease.

Symptoms of prostatitis may include some or all of the following:

- Prostatic symptoms
  - needing to pee often and/or urgently
  - a burning or stinging sensation during urination
  - poor urinary stream or other urinary symptoms

- Throbbing sensations of pain that can radiate to the testes, penis, groin and the lower back areas
- Fever and chills (usually seen with an acute infection only)
- Sometimes a pus-like discharge through the urethra during bowel movements
- Sexual dysfunction and/or loss of libido (sex drive)

These symptoms can be associated with feelings of stress, anxiety and depression. If you have these symptoms see your doctor, who can assess their likely cause and significance.

What Causes It?

Prostatitis can be caused by bacterial infections, viral infections, sexually transmitted infections, inflammation of the urinary tract and other conditions, including stress. Sometimes the cause of prostatitis is unknown. Bacterial infection of the prostate can occur when bugs enter the prostate. This tends to occur suddenly, with sharp, severe symptoms. Men may find urination difficult and extremely painful. It is important to seek treatment promptly as this condition is easy to diagnose.

Chronic prostatitis, sometimes known as chronic pelvic pain syndrome, is the most common form of the disease. It is thought to be due to low-grade inflammation of the prostate gland, sometimes triggered by stress. It is typically difficult to treat and the symptoms tend to recur.

Treatment of Prostatitis

Treatment depends on the underlying cause. For example, antibiotics are used to treat bacterial causes of prostatitis. Sometimes warm baths and anti-inflammatory medication can be helpful. Reassurance that there is no serious underlying cause, such as prostate cancer, for these symptoms can also be helpful for men.

As men get older, two things may happen to their prostates: their prostate can get bigger and/or they can get prostate cancer.

Enlargement of the Prostate or Benign Prostatic Hyperplasia (BPH)

BPH is a non-cancerous condition of ageing, which in some men may cause no more than minimal symptoms. The prostate gland enlarges and may cause problems associated with urination.

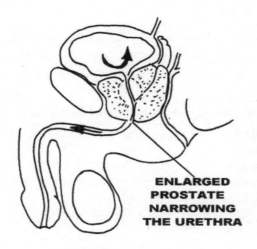

ENLARGED PROSTATE NARROWING THE URETHRA

ENLARGED PROSTATE

What Causes the Prostate to Enlarge?

In normal men, the prostate starts to increase in size, very slowly, from about age 40. The cause of BPH is unknown and is the subject of ongoing research. It is certainly a condition of the ageing male, but we don't know why some men get severe symptoms of BPH while others do not.

There may be genetic factors involved. There may also be dietary factors involved, such as eating a lot of saturated fat and eating only small quantities of fresh fruit. Obesity is associated with more severe BPH symptoms. Regular exercise is thought to protect against BPH, as can moderate amounts of alcohol. The same healthy lifestyle choices for optimal health discussed earlier also seem to apply to this condition.

How Common Is BPH?

Benign enlargement of the prostate is very common and is almost a normal part of ageing. Its incidence rises dramatically as you age.

BPH and Age

Age (Years)	Percentage of Men with BPH
Under 40	Less than 2%
Over 60	50%
Over 85	90%

As you can see above, after a certain age it would be unusual not to have symptoms of an enlarged prostate.

Symptoms and Signs of BPH

You may have BPH and no symptoms whatsoever. However, as the prostate enlarges, it eventually begins to squeeze the urethral tube going through its centre. The common symptoms of BPH can include some or all of the following:

- The need to urinate more frequently
- Nocturia – the inability to sleep through the night without having to get up to urinate. Getting up at night several times to pass urine would not be unusual.
- Urgency – the sudden, intense and sometimes uncontrollable urge to urinate quickly.
- Difficulty in starting urination, also known as hesitancy
- Weak stream – the flow of urine may be slow or weak and urination may be characterised by a repeated start–stop pattern that requires additional straining.
- Terminal dribbling
- Leaking or dribbling of urine. In more severe cases, a patient may develop 'urge incontinence', or the inability to get to the bathroom before losing control of their bladder.
- In severe cases, urine retention can occur, resulting in a complete inability to urinate (this is, however, rare).

These symptoms are known together as 'prostatism'. They can vary widely from one individual to another and men with similar degrees of prostate enlargement may be affected quite differently. This is an important point as ultimately any treatment decision for BPH should be judged on whether the symptoms are affecting your quality of life sufficiently to justify active treatment.

Diagnosis of BPH in its earlier stages can lower the risk of developing complications. The American Urological Association has devised a useful scoring system for BPH. This can help assess the severity of BPH and the need for treatment. It can be a useful monitoring tool to see if your BPH is getting worse over time. Check out the questionnaire on the next page and see how you fare.

Symptom Score for Benign Prostatic Hyperplasia

	Not at all	Less than 1 time in 5	Less than half the time	About half the time	More than half the time	Almost always
1. Over the past month, how often have you had a sensation of not emptying your bladder completely after you finished urinating?	0	1	2	3	4	5
2. Over the past month, how often have you had to urinate again less than two hours after you finished urinating?	0	1	2	3	4	5
3. Over the past month, how often have you found you stopped and started again several times when you urinated?	0	1	2	3	4	5
4. Over the past month, how often have you found it difficult to postpone urination?	0	1	2	3	4	5
5. Over the past month, how often have you had a weak urinary stream?	0	1	2	3	4	5
6. Over the past month, how often have you had to push or strain to begin urination?	0	1	2	3	4	5

(Continued)

(Continued)

	None	1 time	2 times	3 times	4 times	5 or more times
7. Over the past month, how many times did you most typically get up to urinate from the time you went to bed at night until the time you got up in the morning?	0	1	2	3	4	5

Total Symptom Score

Reprinted from the *Journal of Urology* (1992), 148(5), Barry, M.J., Fowler Jr, F.J., O'Leary, M.P., Bruskewitz, R.C., Holtgrewe, H.L., Mebust, W.K. and Cockett, A.T. (The Measurement Committee of the American Urological Association), 'The American Urological Association Symptom Index for Benign Prostatic Hyperplasia', pp. 1549–1557. © American Urological Association, 1992. Reproduced with permission.

Score	Degree of severity of BPH symptoms
1–7	Mild symptoms
8–19	Moderate symptoms
20–25	Severe symptoms

Medical complications from BPH are uncommon. Occasionally it can progress to cause retention of urine but this tends to happen slowly over time. Other recognised complications can include kidney damage, bladder damage, urinary tract infections and bladder stones.

What Can My Doctor Do to Help?

Your doctor can discuss your symptoms with you and help decide on their likely significance. They can help explore your ideas, concerns and expectations. They will look at your medical history and will probably do a prostate exam to evaluate the size and degree of enlargement of the prostate, while at the same time checking for possible infection and cancer. This involves a rectal examination by your doctor using a gloved and lubricated index finger. This allows the prostate to be felt and your doctor can assess its size and also determine whether there are any irregularities on its surface. They may want to do some tests, including analysis of urine and some blood tests to check kidney function. They may also want to do a PSA blood test to rule out prostate cancer.

In more complex cases, your doctor may recommend referral to a urologist for a more detailed assessment and evaluation of your urinary tract. This may include further tests, which may be used to check the prostate and also to examine the rest of the urinary system, including the kidneys and bladder.

Treatment

Options include no active treatment (this is known as watchful waiting), lifestyle measures, herbal remedies including saw palmetto, medication and surgery.

Watchful Waiting

This is a very reasonable option for men who have mild symptoms. Serious complications from BPH are rare. Occasionally it can progress to cause retention of urine but this tends to happen slowly over time.

BPH does not increase the risk of getting prostate cancer. However it can sometimes interfere with the diagnosis of prostate cancer as it can cause the PSA level to increase. The key issue is quality of life. As a man, you need to inform yourself about the pros and cons of active treatment. Educating yourself is the key. Remember, knowledge is power.

Lifestyle Measures

- Simple measures such as restricting fluids in the evening time may help. Make sure you drink enough to stay hydrated (keep your urine clear in colour) and avoid thirst. You should be able to do this and still avoid drinking fluids after 7 p.m.
- Avoid known irritants of the urinary tract. These include alcohol, coffee and spicy foods.
- Review your medications. Some medicines can aggravate prostatic symptoms. These can include antihistamines, some antidepressants, drugs used for bowel spasms and cough bottles containing pseudoephedrine (for example, Sudafed). Diuretics, or 'fluid tablets', can also aggravate these symptoms. If you are taking any of these medications, discuss them with your doctor

to see if they are necessary or if they can be stopped or changed. Don't stop them on your own. While it's great to be a good detective, being your own doctor isn't so smart.

- Avoid eating heavy meals late at night.
- Take regular exercise and follow a good healthy diet. Develop and maintain good sleeping habits.
- Take proactive steps to prevent yourself from falling in the event that you do have to get up at night. Know your way to the bathroom, especially if you are away from home. Identify any potential hazards such as loose carpets and poor lighting and take remedial action. Remember prevention is better than cure, especially when you are talking about a potential broken hip.

What's the Alternative Doc?

Saw palmetto is thought to be a natural remedy for prostatism. It is otherwise known as *Serenoa repens* and is an American dwarf palm plant. The ripe berry of this plant is the source of the herbal extract, which is known to contain a mixture of fatty acids and flavinoids (antioxidants), as well as other substances thought to be good for the prostate. It is not known exactly how saw palmetto works but it appears to be safe. Side effects may include mild nausea or reduced libido but the rate of such problems appears to be much less common than in men taking drugs to treat BPH symptoms. However its long-term safety has not been proven. If saw palmetto does not provide any relief of symptoms after a period of three months then it is reasonable to stop using it.

There has been some suggestion that saw palmetto may affect PSA levels. Therefore, before commencing taking it, it is best to discuss this with your doctor so all the issues relating to your prostate, including the possibility of prostate cancer, can be fully discussed.

<u>Medication</u>

Currently there are two pharmaceutical drug treatment options for BPH. Firstly, alpha blockers can improve BPH symptoms in about 70 per cent of men. These medications relax the smooth muscle of the prostate and bladder neck, which allows urine to flow more easily. These drugs can work quickly to provide relief of symptoms but reverse on stopping the drug. One side effect of alpha blockers is low blood pressure upon standing, which can cause dizziness and light-headedness. Other side effects can include fatigue, headaches and nasal congestion. To minimise these side effects, the dose of medication is usually gradually increased and the first dose is usually given at night. There are several alpha blockers available, all of which can be effective. Examples include terazosin, doxazosin and tamsulosin. The effect of terazosin and doxazosin on blood pressure can be worsened as a result of using medications for erectile dysfunction (ED), such as sildenafil (Viagra), vardenafil (Levitra) and tadalafil (Cialis). These medications should not be used by men who take terazosin or doxazosin. Tamsulosin and alfuzosin do not usually interact with ED medications and can provide a safer alternative option. As with all medication, check with your doctor and pharmacist first.

Secondly, alpha reductase inhibitors (finasteride) work by counter-acting the effects of testosterone within cells of the prostate. By doing so, they may help the prostate from increasing further in size and can sometimes actually shrink the size of the prostate. This can decrease BPH symptoms. Finasteride may take several months to work and it must be used indefinitely to prevent recurrence of symptoms. Up to one-third of men have clinically significant improvements. These drugs tend to be more effective in men with larger prostates. The main side effects are impotence, decreased libido and decreased volume of ejaculate in a small percentage of men. These side effects tend to resolve on stopping the drug. Of note, finasteride tends to lower the PSA (prostate specific antigen) level by about 50 per cent. This is important to realise when screening for prostate cancer. Therefore it is recommended that patients starting finasteride should have a PSA level taken before and six to twelve months after starting therapy.

<u>Surgery</u>

In the past the only effective treatment for BPH was an operation known as a transurethral resection of the prostate (TURP), where the prostate gland was cut and removed or reduced in size. Unfortunately, however, the cure can be worse than the disease. Complications, including impotence, difficulties with ejaculation and problems with urinary continence, can occur, which can raise important issues about a man's quality of life. New forms of minimally invasive prostate surgery are becoming available, including laser surgery. The key issue is to fully understand the risks and benefits of any proposed procedure so that a fully informed decision can be taken. Sometimes the best treatment may be no treatment at all. A decision to undergo surgery should not be taken lightly and reaching one should involve a detailed discussion of the risks and benefits with your urologist.

BPH and Prostate Cancer

BPH can interfere with the diagnosis of prostate cancer as it can cause the PSA level to increase. An increased PSA level does not indicate cancer, but the higher the PSA level the higher the chances of having cancer. Some of the signs of BPH and prostate cancer are the same. However, having BPH does not seem to increase the chances of developing prostate cancer. A man who has BPH may also have undetected prostate cancer at the same time or may develop prostate cancer in the future. Always consult your doctor for more information if you have any concerns in this area.

Prostate Cancer

Prostate cancer is a disease that can affect any man and has no respect for upbringing or address. Irish men have about a one in twelve chance of developing prostate cancer over the course of their lifetime. The vast majority of these cases occur in men over the age of 50. The frequency of prostate cancer is on the rise in Irish men. It has become the most common cancer in men, overtaking lung cancer. With PSA testing on the increase and an ageing population, the incidence of prostate cancer is predicted to rise ahead of breast cancer in women over the next decade.

Prostate cancer differs from most other cancers in the body because small areas of cancer within the prostate are very common and may stay dormant for many years. Most of these cancers grow extremely slowly and so, particularly in elderly men, will never cause any problems. In a small proportion of men, the prostate cancer does grow more quickly and in some cases may spread to other parts of the body, particularly the bones.

What Are the Risk Factors for Developing Prostate Cancer?

We do not yet know exactly what causes prostate cancer, but we do know that certain risk factors are linked to the disease. Some risk factors, such as smoking, can be eliminated by simply quitting (or better again not starting in the first place). Others, like a person's age or family history, can't be changed. But having a risk factor, or even several, doesn't mean that you will get a particular disease. Many people with one or more risk factors never get cancer, while others with this disease may have had no known risk factors.

As well as increasing age, there are a number of recognised risk factors for prostate cancer:

- Family history – your risk of prostate cancer increases if there is a history of prostate cancer in your family.
- Nationality – prostate cancer is much more prevalent in the Western world than, for example, in Asia. However, research has shown that Asians who come to live in the West also develop a high risk of prostate cancer. This has led many researchers to focus on dietary risk factors.
- Diet – a diet high in saturated fat, namely animal fat, is associated with a significantly increased risk of prostate cancer. The high-saturated-fat diet of the Western world is thought to be one of the main reasons why prostate cancer is so much higher in the West than in places like Asia where much less saturated fat and animal fat is eaten. There is considerable research being undertaken looking at diet and other supplements that can help prevent prostate cancer. While the results of research studies are not yet clear, you may be able to reduce your risk of prostate cancer by changing the way you eat. Eating less red meat and fat and eating more vegetables, fruits and wholegrains may help lower your risk for other types of cancer, as well as other diseases.

It should be mentioned that vasectomy and BPH are not associated with an increased risk of prostate cancer.

The Prostate Diet

There are currently a number of foodstuffs rich in antioxidants (substances that have cancer-preventing properties) that are thought to help prevent prostate cancer. You will notice that there is a good deal of crossover here with heart disease prevention and general wellness. Nevertheless, I have put some of these together and labelled them as the 'prostate diet'.

Tomatoes

Tomatoes appear to be out on their own as far as prostate cancer prevention is concerned. Tomatoes, pink grapefruit, watermelon and apricots are rich in a powerful antioxidant known as lycopene that helps prevent damage to DNA and may help lower prostate cancer risk. People who have diets rich in tomatoes appear to have a lower risk of certain types of cancer, especially cancer of the prostate. Other potential benefits of lycopenes include a lower risk of heart disease, lower levels of LDL (bad) cholesterol (see Chapter 6), less macular degeneration (a disease of the eyes that can lead to blindness), and strengthening of the immune system.

Tomatoes are the best food source of lycopene. Tomato-based products such as tomato juice, puree and pastes, canned tomatoes and cooked tomatoes may be even better than raw tomatoes, as lycopene becomes concentrated in cooked or processed tomatoes; pizza and pasta lovers take note. Lycopene from eating fruit and vegetables has no known side effects as long as you are not allergic to these foods. Very large quantities of tomato-based products taken over a long period of time can give the skin an orange colour, however.

Other dietary sources that can reduce the risk of prostate cancer include:

- A diet rich in fresh fruit and vegetables, particularly green leafy vegetables like broccoli, spinach and cabbage
- Plenty of dietary sources of Vitamins A, C and E
- Wholegrain cereals
- Nuts and seeds, which are rich in Vitamin E and contain alpha-Linolenic acid (an omega-3 fatty acid)

- Selenium – a mineral with strong antioxidant properties. Natural dietary sources of selenium include Brazil nuts, fish, garlic, poultry and meat. Grains and vegetables grown in selenium-rich soil are also an excellent source of this mineral.
- Vitamin D, which is activated in our skin by exposure to ultraviolet light
- Vitamin E – a powerful antioxidant and may be protective
- Oily fish – particularly fish from deep cold waters, which are rich in omega-3 fatty acids. We know this is good for your heart, but it also looks like omega-3 fatty acids are good for your prostate.
- Soy-based products such as soy milk and tofu
- Zinc is also good for the prostate – oysters, soy, nuts, wheat germ, bran, eggs, pumpkin seeds and lentils are full of it.

It's always a good idea to check with your doctor about taking vitamins or supplements before you start to do so. Natural dietary sources of vitamins and minerals are preferable to taking supplements. As well as eating plenty of the listed foods that are good for you, it is important to stay away from the bad stuff. In this case I mean saturated fat, red meat and processed foods.

Signs and Symptoms of Prostate Cancer

One of the problems related to prostate cancer is that, in its early stages, it often does not have symptoms. When symptoms do occur, they may include any of the following:

- Having a sense of urgency, a need to rush to the toilet to pass urine
- Passing urine more often and/or at night
- Difficulty getting the flow of urine started (hesitancy)
- Starting and stopping whilst passing urine (a poor stream)
- Discomfort (pain or burning) while passing urine

- A feeling of not having emptied the bladder fully
- Dribbling of urine at the end
- Blood in the urine or semen
- Pain or stiffness in the back, hips or pelvis

Of course, these symptoms can be caused by many other conditions, including a urinary tract infection, BPH or even simple wear and tear arthritis in the case of back stiffness. The prostate enlarges as men get older, and most men have some symptoms affecting urination. However, if you have these symptoms, it is important to go to your doctor so they can be properly evaluated. There is little to be gained from sticking your head in the sand, yet there is good evidence that many men do delay seeking medical help, often to their cost.

Diagnosis of Prostate Cancer

Early diagnosis of prostate cancer is important for successful treatment. None of the following tests is an individually conclusive indicator of prostate cancer. Your doctor is likely to use more than one test to determine whether or not you are affected by prostate cancer.

<u>Rectal Examination</u>

Your doctor can actually feel the size of the prostate gland by doing a rectal examination with a gloved finger, which allows him/her to feel your prostate. This can help tell if it is enlarged and/or if there are any suspicious-feeling bumps or irregularities on the prostate. However, an enlarged prostate does not, on its own, indicate prostate cancer.

<u>The PSA Test</u>

This is a blood test that measures the amount of prostate specific antigen (PSA) in the bloodstream. PSA is a substance produced in the prostate gland that helps to liquefy semen. Some PSA can also get into the bloodstream, which is why measuring the level of PSA can be a marker of prostate health. A raised PSA level can be the first indicator of otherwise asymptomatic prostate cancer. However, while a high reading suggests prostate cancer, the PSA test is not specific for cancer and raised levels can occur because of benign enlargement or inflammation of the prostate gland.

The PSA test is the best way to detect prostate cancer in its early stage. Traditionally, PSA levels of zero to four were considered normal. It is now recognised that PSA levels tend to rise with age so age-adjusted PSA levels are suggested. The table below shows the upper limits of acceptable PSA levels in the bloodstream, adjusted by age.

Age-Adjusted PSA Levels

Age (Years)	PSA Cut Off (ng/mL)
50–59	≥3.0
60–69	≥4.0
70 and over	>5.0

So far so good; shouldn't we all have this test done? Well, if you have symptoms that indicate possible prostate cancer, such as urinary prostatic symptoms, weight loss, backache or abnormal findings on rectal examination, then the answer is most definitely yes – a PSA test can help in the diagnosis. However, for the man who has no symptoms the answer is not so clearcut. The problem is that not all men with a raised PSA level will have prostate cancer so these men may be subjected to unnecessary follow-up tests, including prostate biopsy, and all the potential anxiety that these can generate, as well as potential side effects from an invasive procedure.

Research suggests that many men with a raised PSA will not have any prostate cancer in their biopsy. On the other hand, some men with prostate cancer will have a normal PSA result.

In addition, prostate cancer has a long dormant phase and this means that cancer cells can exist in the prostate for many years without causing any harm, and sometimes will never cause any harm. Prostate cancer is one of those conditions that older men can die with, but not necessarily from. This is a big potential difference between prostate cancer and many other cancers. However, sometimes prostate cancer can be more aggressive and spread to other parts of the body, especially the bones.

Other conditions that can cause a raised PSA reading include benign enlargement of the prostate (BPH) and inflammation and/or infection of the prostate. Ejaculation can cause a temporary rise in the PSA level, peaking after about an hour and returning to base line after a period of 24 to 48 hours. Therefore, it is recommended not to perform a PSA test if you have an active urinary tract infection or if you have ejaculated in the previous 48 hours.

Research is ongoing as to whether PSA testing should be used to routinely screen every man for prostate cancer. Many medical professionals feel it wrong to introduce national screening in this country because the effectiveness of screening is currently unproven and the side effects of treatment can be significant. At the moment the potential benefits from PSA screening remain unproven and the jury is still out. Two large international trials are currently underway to try to answer this important question. The results of these trials hopefully will provide more clarity around this complex issue. Information is power. By educating yourself about your own bodily functions you are in the best position to appreciate any changes. You have the right to have a PSA test done if you request it. The main thing to understand is that it is not a black and white issue. Discuss any areas of concern with your family doctor. He or she can help you make an informed decision about what is best for your health.

<u>Other Tests</u>

Further tests on the prostate can be carried out by a specialist in the area (a urologist). These can include:

- An ultrasound scan – a small probe is inserted into the back passage and a scan taken to show the exact size of the prostate gland.
- A prostate biopsy – a small probe can be inserted into the back passage and a tiny sample of prostate tissue can be removed and analysed.
- A bone scan – a scan of the bones can be taken to see if the cancer has spread to the bones near the prostate.

Treatment Options for Prostate Cancer

This is an area that is the subject of ongoing research. There are a number of treatment options that can be taken singly or sometimes in combination. All of these treatments have pluses and minuses. It is important to inform yourself fully about all the options, including the option of 'watchful waiting', i.e. simply keeping an eye on your prostate. This can be a very reasonable option as many men with prostate cancer do not have aggressive forms of the condition and their condition grows so slowly that no active treatment is needed.

The decision to have active treatment and which type of treatment to undergo is an important decision that you should take in conjunction with your specialist, as side effects from these treatments can be significant. Surgery, radiotherapy and hormone therapy all have different side effects that need to be considered. These side effects include urinary incontinence, reduced ejaculation, lowered sex drive and long-term impotence, as well as hot flushes, tiredness and sweats.

Options include surgery, radiotherapy, hormone therapy or a combination of these treatments:

- Surgical removal of the entire prostate is known as a 'radical prostatectomy'. Complications from this can include impotence and urinary incontinence.
- Radiotherapy can include either external beam radiotherapy, where the prostate is irradiated from outside the body, or more recently an option of placing small radioactive seeds into the prostate, which irradiate it from the inside out.
- Hormone treatment can lower the testosterone levels (this is like giving the patient the male menopause). Drugs can be used to lower the level of testosterone in the blood, which has the effect of slowing or stopping the growth of the cancerous tumour. However, some prostate tumours develop the ability to grow without testosterone.

Research is ongoing into other potential treatments for prostate cancer. One such option may be a new drug called abiraterone. Early research suggests that this drug can shrink the prostate in men with prostate cancer. Large scale trials will be needed comparing this treatment to established treatment options to see if it really is a step forward.

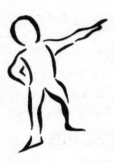

Key Points

- The prostate is an important gland for a man's sexual health.
- Many men lack knowledge and information about the prostate gland.
- Disorders of the prostate gland, especially benign enlargement (BPH), are common, especially as men get older.
- Be aware of the symptoms of prostate problems.
- Prostate cancer is the most common cancer in men and is on the increase.
- Often this cancer can be very slow-growing and difficult to diagnose.
- The PSA blood test, when raised, can be an early marker of prostate cancer.
- At present the jury is still out on the benefits of screening for prostate cancer.
- Stay informed about your prostate health and discuss this issue with your doctor.

9

When It Won't Stay Up – Erectile Dysfunction (Impotence)

 The inability to achieve and maintain an adequate erection for satisfactory sexual performance is extremely common and probably affects most men at some stage in their lives.

This important men's health issue is called erectile dysfunction (ED). The word 'impotence' is derived from the Latin for 'loss of power' and implies a complete inability to get an erection. The term 'erectile dysfunction' is preferred because there is a whole variety of erection-related problems. For some men this is only a temporary effect, perhaps when they are under stress, tired or have drunk too much alcohol; for others it can be a more long-lasting problem. However, ED can be an early sign of damage to the blood vessels elsewhere in the body, for example, the heart, the brain or the legs. It can have a significant impact on the quality of life for a man, his partner and their relationship.

What Is the Cause of Erectile Dysfunction?

There is no easy answer to this as there may be several different factors involved. We do know that many men still suffer needlessly in silence, as they either feel too embarrassed to raise the issue or they feel it is part of 'normal ageing'. Fortunately, these types of issues are no longer taboo and have benefited from a great deal of media exposure in recent years. This has been helped enormously by the arrival of effective medical treatments for this condition, such as Viagra. As a result, men should have the confidence to discuss this important health issue with their family doctor and get appropriate help and treatment.

How Common Is Erectile Dysfunction?

It can occur at any age but is more common as a man gets older. About 50 per cent of all men aged between 40 and 70 and about 70 per cent of men aged over 70 are affected by erectile dysfunction issues.

How Normal Erections Work

Knowledge of how an erection works can be helpful in understanding the causes of erectile dysfunction (ED) as well as the treatment options. Normal erections require healthy arteries, veins and nerves, a mind that is 'tuned in', enough testosterone in the system and a chemical called nitric oxide. It is a complex process that starts with physical arousal or erotic thoughts. Penile erection is usually triggered by one of two main mechanisms: direct stimulation of the genitalia or stimuli coming from the brain (fantasy, smell, etc.). This causes messages in the form of chemicals (nitric oxide) to go from the brain down the spinal cord to the penis. The penis is an organ with spongy erectile tissue composed predominantly of muscle. These chemicals then cause the penis to enlarge by increasing its blood supply. This increased blood flow into and storage of blood within the spongy erectile tissue of the penis leads to an increase in its pressure and the development of rigidity (hardness). The increased pressure of blood in the penis helps to prevent blood from escaping out of the penis. Ongoing sexual arousal results in more chemicals going from the brain via the spinal cord into the nerve endings of the penis. Both of these processes help to maintain the erection.

The erection mechanism can be compared to blowing up a balloon. In this analogy the balloon is the penis, which needs a rapid increase in blood flow to become erect. The knot on the balloon represents the valve structure in the penis that keeps the penis erect. A firm balloon depends on being able to blow air quickly into it. A knot or pressure in place prevents the air from getting back out and keeps the balloon firm. If sexual stimulation ceases, then the balloon will lose its air and deflate. Alternatively, if stimulation continues, more and more air will enter the balloon until it eventually bursts (this represents orgasm).

When It Goes Wrong

Medical conditions such as heart disease or diabetes can physically damage the arteries and nerves involved in erections. They can do this by causing narrowing of the penile artery, which prevents proper blood flow, or scarring of the spongy erection tissue, which prevents proper trapping of blood. Psychological issues such as anxiety or depression can prevent the nitric oxide from reaching the level required to induce erection.

Physical Causes of Erectile Dysfunction

Erectile dysfunction has an underlying physical cause in 80 per cent of men with the problem. Erectile dysfunction can cause anxiety, loss of self-esteem and loss of confidence, which can make the situation worse.

Your ED is likely to be physical in cause if:

- You have a normal sex drive (libido)
- You don't get night-time or early morning erections
- The onset is gradual over time
- You have normal ejaculation
- You have other risk factors for damage to the blood vessels, such as smoking, high blood pressure and high cholesterol levels

Narrowing of the Penile Artery

This is the most common physical cause. Narrowing of the blood vessel (artery) supplying the penis is due to fatty plaques sticking to the sides of the artery causing, in effect, the pipes to become furred up. This condition is known as atherosclerosis and can occur gradually over many years. It is responsible for heart disease, stroke and poor circulation to the legs as well as erectile dysfunction. So, developing erectile dysfunction may be the first sign of narrowings of blood vessels elsewhere in the body. The penile artery is 3 millimetres in diameter and the coronary artery supplying the heart is only 5 millimetres in diameter. Erectile dysfunction can be an early warning sign of potentially serious future health problems. Don't ignore it.

The risk of developing atherosclerosis and erectile dysfunction is increased by these factors:

- Smoking – this can damage the lining of the blood vessels anywhere in the body and the penile artery is no exception. Smoking can double your chances of getting ED.
- Diabetes
- High blood pressure
- High cholesterol and blood fat levels

- Family history of heart disease or stroke
- Metabolic syndrome

Obesity

Being obese is associated with an increased risk of ED, probably due to the effects of obesity on blood sugar levels and circulation.

Alcohol and Other Drugs

Alcohol is a good servant and a bad master. As we know, it is a depressant and certainly more than a few units of alcohol at any one time can impede performance. This has been described in medical circles as 'brewer's droop', where one has an inability to maintain an erection after a few drinks. This, of course, can cause subsequent anxiety about performance on future occasions, even when alcohol has not been consumed.

Chronic alcohol abuse can cause liver damage, which raises the level of oestrogen (the female hormone) in the body, thereby causing impotence. However, alcohol in moderation can help protect against erectile dysfunction.

Other illegal drugs, including cocaine and marijuana, can cause sexual dysfunction. Just like chronic alcohol abuse, marijuana can raise the levels of oestrogen in the body, thereby causing impotence.

Diabetes

Erectile dysfunction is very commonly seen in men with diabetes. Diabetes can affect the nerve supply to the penis as well as narrowing the penile artery. If you have diabetes, it is extremely important, not just for your sexual health but for the general health of your blood vessels, to keep your blood sugar levels tightly controlled, not to smoke, to keep your blood pressure optimal, to take regular exercise and to keep your cholesterol and weight at acceptable levels.

Disorders of the Nervous System

As mentioned above, diabetes can affect the nerve supply to the penis, which can result in ED. Other conditions, such as multiple sclerosis, damage to the spinal cord, including spinal surgery, stroke and other forms of nerve damage can also cause impotence in this manner.

Cycling

Cycling, particularly long-distance cycling, has been associated with ED, probably due to a pressure effect of the saddle on the nerves that supply the penis.

Hormones

Hormonal causes of erectile dysfunction are uncommon and include testosterone deficiency. This is generally associated with loss of libido.

The Ageing Process

Erectile dysfunction becomes more common as we age. While our male testosterone levels do tend to reduce as we get older, they generally remain within the normal range, even for many elderly men. So, it is not the ageing process per se that causes erectile dysfunction, rather it is ageing of the blood vessels. This is caused by medical conditions such as diabetes or atherosclerosis, as discussed above. Also, as we get older there is a higher chance that we will be on medication for various conditions. The medication in itself maybe the culprit when it comes to erectile dysfunction. The classical example of erectile dysfunction caused by medication is the beta blocker, which has widely been used to treat high blood pressure and palpitations.

Medications That Can Cause Erectile Dysfunction

- Antidepressants
- Beta blockers
- Some diuretics or 'water tablets'
- Anti-ulcer drugs such as cimetidine
- Diazepam (Valium) and other sedatives
- Some drugs used to treat epilepsy
- Antihistamines
- Drugs used to treat high blood pressure

Psychological Causes of Erectile Dysfunction

Many mental health issues can cause erectile dysfunction. These include stress, anxiety and depression, as well as relationship difficulties. Anxiety and depression can result from erectile dysfunction as well, so it can be a chicken-and-egg situation. A psychological cause for ED is more likely if:

- You can still get some erections, for example, early morning erections or erections when masturbating.
- The onset of ED is sudden.
- There is loss of sex drive (libido).
- There is premature ejaculation or failure to ejaculate.
- There are relationship problems or other major stresses.

Psychological causes of erectile dysfunction can occur when we are under excess stress or when we are feeling very anxious or indeed are suffering from depression. In all these situations our body and mind are out of balance. Erectile dysfunction may occur as a result. A classical example of this is performance anxiety, where the worry or fear of not being able to perform or maintain an erection causes such intense anxiety that the erection process is blocked or inhibited.

173

Needless to say, there is a cause-and-effect process here also, in that erectile dysfunction from any cause can result in profound anxiety and a loss of confidence and self-esteem for many men.

It is normal for men to get night-time and early morning erections. If you still have these then it is likely your erectile dysfunction may have a psychological basis. The absence of night-time or early morning erections suggests a physical cause of erectile dysfunction.

What Can I Do if I Have ED?

Your doctor can make an informed decision about the likely causes of your erectile dysfunction from a good chat with you and an appropriate assessment, which may include a physical examination and blood tests. Don't let embarrassment or fear prevent you from taking action and seeking help. If you have any concerns or questions about your sexual health, ask. Your doctor is there to help you but don't leave it up to your doctor to raise these important issues.

Tests for Erectile Dysfunction

Tests carried out may include:

- Blood tests after a period of fasting to check the blood sugar level (for diabetes) and also to measure cholesterol and blood fat levels
- Blood pressure test
- ECG and/or other heart tests
- Other blood tests such as checking your testosterone levels

Most men presenting with erectile dysfunction do not require any further tests, but a minority may benefit from more specialised tests with a urologist.

Treatment of ED

Treatment depends on the underlying cause of ED. Key areas that can help include maintaining a healthy lifestyle, looking after your mental health, examining your current medication, pelvic floor exercises, drug therapy, injection therapy, urethral suppositories, vacuum devices and surgery.

Healthy Lifestyle

There is good evidence that following a healthy lifestyle can really help with erectile dysfunction. A heart-healthy diet, taking plenty of exercise and watching your stress levels can all help keep you in good shape. It is important to keep your weight down and avoid tobacco products.

A regular medical check-up will help ensure your blood pressure, cholesterol and blood sugar levels are well controlled. While taking a tablet like Viagra can help cure erectile dysfunction it won't necessarily address the underlying health issues. It is no substitute for the healthy foundations we all need for good long-term health.

Mental Health

It is important to optimise your mental well-being. This includes recognising and treating any underlying depression or anxiety and moderating your alcohol intake. Assess your level of stress. Do you cope well under pressure? Have you enough down time? Counselling can be helpful, particularly if there are relationship issues. Sex therapy can sometimes play an important role. This works best when the patient is well motivated and has the time to invest in the process.

Reviewing Your Medication

It can be useful to review your medication carefully with your doctor or pharmacist. If your doctor thinks some of your medications may be the culprit he may decide to stop one medication at a time for a few weeks to see what benefit it has. It is important not to stop medication without consulting your doctor as this may have health consequences. It's okay to be a good detective but not your own doctor. Talk to your doctor, he or she is there to help you.

Pelvic Floor Exercises

These are exercises to strengthen your pelvic floor and can sometimes help with ED. They involve the muscles you use to stop yourself from passing wind and also those muscles used to stop the flow of urine. A physiotherapist would be able to give you a leaflet to help with this.

Medical Treatment

This has been revolutionised over the past ten years or so since the arrival of drugs like Viagra. The impact of these drugs has been massive, not just because they work but also because they have done so much to increase awareness of ED as a health issue. Early media coverage generated massive worldwide demand for this medication. Prescribing drugs like Viagra is now mainstream medical practice and there is no need to be embarrassed or shy about asking your doctor if you might benefit. At least it gives you an opportunity for this important health issue to be discussed in a sensitive and confidential manner.

There are three different types of drug available at present:

- Viagra (sildenafil)
- Cialis (tadalafil)
- Levitra (varenafil)

How Do They Work?

They all work slightly differently but all affect hormonal chemicals that come from the brain during sexual arousal. These drugs work by increasing the amount of nitric oxide produced. This chemical does two important things: it causes the nerve connections between the brain and the penis to become more fine-tuned; and it also increases the blood supply to the penis and causes the blood vessels in the penis to widen, causing an erection. These drugs in themselves do not create erections but they make an erection much more likely after sexual arousal. Ideally they should be taken about an hour before sexual activity and the effects can last several hours.

Do They Work?

Yes, in the majority of cases (about 70–80 per cent) these drugs can produce a good erection. Some men may find that one drug works and another doesn't so it can be a trial-and-error process. Also, the dosage may vary. However, these medications can produce a good erection even when the blood supply to the penis is narrowed, as in cases of atherosclerosis and nerve damage, for example.

Do They Have any Side Effects?

Like all medicine there is a potential risk of side effects. Discuss this with your doctor. Common side effects include headache, facial flushing, nasal congestion and stomach upset. About 3 per cent of men who take Viagra get visual disturbances, most commonly affecting colour vision. This is often described as a bluish tinge.

It is felt that Viagra is generally safe to take for men with heart disease, provided their condition is stable and well-controlled. Discuss this further with your doctor if you have concerns.

Do They Interact with Other Medicines?

There is a risk of severe interaction with nitrates (used in patients with heart disease and angina) and for this reason drugs like Viagra cannot be taken if you are on nitrates. Check with your doctor or pharmacist about other potential interactions. The effectiveness of some of these drugs is affected if taken after a fatty meal – another good reason to watch your diet.

Injection Therapy

An injection of a drug called Caverject with a very fine needle is made into the penis, which usually causes an erection to occur within about 15 minutes that can last up to an hour. While this can sound scary, most men can learn the technique. The erection occurs even if you are not sexually aroused (unlike medication).

Side effects can include penile pain and discomfort. A rarer side effect of this injection is a prolonged painful erection, which is known as priapism. This condition needs emergency treatment to prevent long-term damage to the penis.

Injection treatment is less popular now that oral medication is available, for obvious reasons.

Urethral Pellet

An urethral suppository (brand name Muse) is a pellet, the size of a grain of rice, that is placed in the tip of the urethra. An erection usually occurs within 10 minutes and can last up to 60 minutes, though this can vary from person to person. This treatment is based on the finding that the urethra (the tube in the penis through which urine and semen flow) can absorb certain medications into the surrounding tissues, creating an erection. Muse urethral suppositories use the same medication as is used in injection therapy.

Vacuum Devices

The penis is put into an airtight plastic container and a hand-held pump is then used to pump air out of the container to create a vacuum. This causes blood to flow into the penis, leading to an erection in about 80 per cent of men within a few minutes. A special band is then put around the base of the erect penis to keep the blood in the penis until after intercourse. The band is then removed and the penis becomes limp. Side effects can include penile pain and bruising.

Penile Surgery

This can be an option for some men in which a surgeon inserts a rod or prosthesis permanently into the penis. There are two types of device. A rigid one uses a silicone rod that can be bent up and down; it keeps the penis erect at all times. There is also an inflatable option, which has an inbuilt pump to cause an erection.

Aphrodisiacs

These are substances that are reputed to improve virility. For many years various foods and herbs have been promoted as having sexual vitality properties. Examples include oysters, ginger and chocolate. Whether or not they work is certainly very difficult, if not impossible, to prove scientifically. However the placebo effect can have a strong influence on us. If we believe something is going to work then there is a good chance it just might. It is best to be cautious about taking any herbs or supplements. Make sure to discuss this first with your doctor, especially if you are already on prescribed medication.

Self-Assessment Questionnaire

The following self-assessment questionnaire on erectile dysfunction can help in terms of defining the nature of the problem. It has been designed as an easy-to-use diagnostic tool to help the assessment of both the presence and severity of ED. Each question has five possible responses. Circle the number that best describes your own situation. Select only one answer to each question.

IIEF-5 Scoring System

Over the past six months:

	1	2	3	4	5
How do you rate your *confidence* that you could get and keep an erection?	Very low	Low	Moderate	High	Very high
When you had erections with sexual stimulation, *how often* were your erections hard enough for penetration?	Almost never/never	A few times (much less than half the time)	Sometimes (about half the time)	Most times (much more than half the time)	Almost always/always
During sexual intercourse, *how often* were you able to maintain your erection after you had penetrated (entered) your partner?	Almost never/never	A few times (much less than half the time)	Sometimes (about half the time)	Most times (much more than half the time)	Almost always/always
During sexual intercourse, *how difficult* was it to maintain your erection to the completion of intercourse?	Extremely difficult	Very difficult	Difficult	Slightly difficult	Not difficult
When you attempted sexual intercourse, *how often* was it satisfactory for you?	Almost never/never	A few times (much less than half the time)	Sometimes (about half the time)	Most times (much more than half the time)	Almost always/always

The IIEF-5 score is the sum of questions 1 to 5. The lowest possible score is 5 and the highest possible score 25.

Reprinted with permission from Macmillan Publishers Ltd: *International Journal of Impotence Research*, 'Development and Evaluation of an Abridged, 5-item Version of the International Index of Erectile Function (IIEF-5) as a Diagnostic Tool for Erectile Dysfunction', Rosen, R.C., Cappelleri, J.C., Smith, M.D., Lipsky, J. and Pena, B.M. (Table 2) (1999) 11(6), 319–326, © 1999.

How Did You Fare?

Key:

Score	Result
22–25	No ED
17–21	Mild ED
12–16	Mild to moderate ED
8–11	Moderate ED
5–7	Severe ED

If a man scores 21 or less, then his chance of truly having erectile dysfunction rises to about 93 per cent. If he scores 22 or more, then it falls to 2 per cent or less.

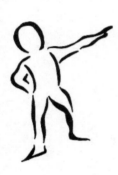

Key Points

- Erectile dysfunction is an important and common men's health issue.
- ED can be an early warning sign of damage to the circulation, for example, from smoking or high cholesterol.
- Our sexual health can be closely related to our sense of physical and mental well-being.
- ED can often be effectively treated.
- If you have a problem, don't be embarrassed to talk to your doctor about ED.

10

Male Infertility

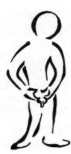

The normal male fertility process involves being able to make enough mature sperm of the right size and shape and get those sperm to reach and fertilise the egg, thereby achieving pregnancy. In general, men reach their peak fertility levels at about the age of 25 and fertility levels start to decline after the age of 40. However, many men can remain fertile right up until the age of 80 and beyond.

Male fertility requires many complex biological conditions to be met, including:

- The ability to have and maintain an erection
- Having enough sperm of the right shape that move in the right way
- Having enough semen to carry the sperm to the egg

The issue of male infertility is a sensitive one for men and their partners. The psychological impact of infertility upon individuals or couples affected by it may be significant. It can result in distress, anxiety, relationship difficulties and possibly depression.

183

Infertility for a couple is commonly defined as the failure to achieve pregnancy after regular unprotected sex for at least a year. Some couples have never been able to conceive – this is known as primary infertility. Secondary infertility describes couples who have previously been pregnant at least once, but have not been able to achieve another pregnancy.

How Common Is Infertility?

Male infertility is common. About one in six couples attempting their first pregnancy meet with disappointment. The cause of infertility tends to follow the rule of thirds. Approximately, the problem is with the male one-third of the time, with the female one-third of the time and with both one-third of the time. Therefore the male is at least partly responsible in about 50 per cent of all cases of infertile couples.

Sperm Development

The production of sperm is known medically as spermatogenesis. This process occurs in the ducts and tubes of the testes. Cell division there produces mature sperm cells known as spermatozoa. These sperm cells contain one half of a man's genetic code. The process of sperm development takes about eighty days to produce a mature sperm from start to finish. Therefore any illness or infection a man may have had at the start of the cycle may still affect sperm production two or three months later, even if he is well at the time of examination.

The Temperature of Sperm

Sperm are produced better and survive longer in a low-temperature environment. This is the main reason why the testes are outside the body. For this reason you should be cautious about wearing any clothing, such as very tight-fitting underpants or trousers, or activities – such as excessive use of saunas or steam-rooms – that can increase the temperature of sperm. Sitting on a bicycle saddle can also have an adverse effect on sperm production, particularly if you are wearing tight-fitting shorts.

Causes of Infertility

Causes of infertility include a wide range of physical as well as emotional factors. Approximately one-third to a half of all infertility is due to a 'male' factor. A 'female' factor – scarring from sexually transmitted infection or endometriosis, ovulation dysfunction, poor nutrition, hormone imbalance, ovarian cysts, pelvic infection, tumour, or transport system abnormality from the cervix through the fallopian tubes – is responsible for 40–50 per cent of infertility in couples. The remaining 10–30 per cent of infertility cases may be caused by contributing factors from both partners, or no cause may be identified.

Increased risk for infertility can be associated with the following conditions and factors in men:

- Varicoceles (see the Chapter 12 for a description of this)
- Undescended testes
- Retrograde ejaculation
- Poor sperm development
- Infections
- Medication
- Recreational drug use
- Chronic medical conditions
- Trauma
- Lifestyle factors
- Testosterone deficiency

Undescended Testes

This affects nearly 1 per cent of males. Our testes start to develop high up in our belly area and have usually come down, or 'descended', by the time we are born. However, if they fail to descend they are known as undescended testes. This increases the lifelong risk of testicular cancer. For this reason undescended testes are always 'brought down' surgically into the scrotal sac if they have not descended themselves by the age of two.

However, despite this, men with a history of undescended testes still have reduced fertility, even when it is one-sided. This is because it appears that there is reduced ability to produce sperm levels in both the normally descended and the undescended testis.

Retrograde Ejaculation

This results from failure of the bladder neck to close during ejaculation so that sperm goes up into the bladder instead of out through the penis. Clues to this condition may include cloudy urine after ejaculation or reduced or even 'dry' ejaculation. It may result from bladder surgery or a disease that affects the nervous system.

Infections

Mumps infection can cause swelling and inflammation of the testicles. This is known as orchitis and can have a long-term effect on sperm levels and fertility. Mumps orchitis is usually one-sided but sometimes it can affect both testicles. A complication of this condition is that the testicles can shrink and waste away. Other infections that can affect fertility include sexually transmitted infections, such as chlamydia, and infections like E. coli in the semen, which can affect sperm motility (movement). General infections of the body can also temporarily affect sperm production and lead to reduced fertility.

Steroids

Steroids, which are used to treat conditions such as arthritis and asthma, can lead to an increased steroid level in the blood, which can reduce the ability of the body to make sperm. This is usually reversible on reducing or stopping the steroid. Some medical conditions such as Cushing's disease can result in the body making too much steroid.

Anabolic steroids are sometimes taken illegally by athletes and body-builders in the form of supplements. These are highly dangerous for long-term health. Not only will they affect fertility but they can also, amongst other things, cause heart attacks and liver cancer.

Other medications that can sometimes affect fertility include anti-cancer drugs like chemotherapy, some antifungal drugs, cimetidine (used to treat stomach ulcers), spironolactone (used to treat heart failure) and medications to treat high blood pressure.

Recreational Drugs

Many illegal drugs affect fertility levels in many different ways. These include the usual suspects of cigarettes and alcohol, as well as marijuana and others. This can be a reversible process, which is yet another good reason to adopt a healthy lifestyle.

Chronic Medical Conditions

Chronic medical conditions can be associated with infertility. These include diabetes, haemochromatosis, kidney disease, liver disease, high fevers, infections, cystic fibrosis and sickle-cell anaemia.

Trauma

Testicular injury can impair the ability of the testes to work properly. Examples would include trauma to the scrotal area and testicular torsion (discussed in Chapter 12).

Lifestyle Factors

Lifestyle factors, including smoking cigarettes, poor diet, excess alcohol, obesity and lack of exercise, can affect fertility levels. Wearing tight trousers or underpants can increase the temperature of the testes and result in reduced fertility. Environmental toxins or pollutants can also potentially be a factor in male infertility.

Testosterone Deficiency

Testosterone plays an important part in sperm development and a lack of testosterone in the system can lead to a low sperm count. Disorders of the pituitary gland in the brain can also cause testosterone deficiency. These disorders include an over- or under-active thyroid, haemochromatosis and Cushing's disease, as well as tumours of the pituitary gland.

Genetic or Chromosomal Defects

Some genetic or chromosomal defects can affect the development of the genitals. While most men have one X (female) and one Y (male) chromosome, certain disorders add an extra chromosome to our genetic make-up, with many different consequences.

The most common of these disorders is known as *Klinefelter's syndrome*, which affects about one in every 500 males. In this condition, there is an extra X chromosome. Characteristically these men have abnormal breast enlargement (known as gynaecomastia), smaller-than-normal testes, sparse facial and body hair, and no sperm production. There is also delayed onset of other secondary sexual characteristics such as deepening of the voice and development of the genitals.

Another chromosomal disorder is known as *XYY syndrome*, whereby the affected man has an extra Y chromosome. This again affects about one in every 500 men. These men tend to be very tall, some have had severe acne and some have a tendency to antisocial behaviour. While some of these men have no sperm, some produce normal amounts of sperm.

The extremely rare v*anishing testes syndrome* affects about one in every 20,000 males; these unfortunate men are born without testicles.

Kallman's syndrome is another rare cause of infertility. It occurs in only one in every ten thousand men. It is often associated with loss of smell, deafness, cleft lip and palate, kidney problems and colour blindness as well as infertility.

Other Causes of Infertility

Male infertility may also be caused by sexual dysfunctions, such as premature ejaculation, reduced libido and erectile dysfunction. This may be due to low testosterone levels resulting from an underlying condition. These are all potentially reversible causes of infertility.

Some men have infertility for which there is no known cause at present. In addition, some known causes of infertility do not have any treatments.

Research is ongoing into this important men's health area. As knowledge and understanding increases, more causes and, hopefully, treatments will be discovered.

Investigating Fertility Issues in Men

Talking to your doctor is a good place to start. He or she can check your medical history and any risk factors for infertility. Your doctor can discuss your ideas, concerns and expectations. A physical examination to check your testes and to see if you have a varicocele in your scrotum is important. The next step usually would be to arrange a sperm test.

Semen Analysis – Checking a Sperm Sample

Semen analysis is a test used to evaluate male fertility. This test, also called a sperm count, measures the amount and quality of seminal fluid or ejaculate. Seminal fluid contains male reproductive cells (semen or sperm) and normally is expelled through the penis during ejaculation (sexual climax; orgasm).

This is a highly accurate test. However, it is worth noting that a normal result does not guarantee fertility, as fertility is naturally a couple-related phenomenon. However, a normal result is certainly reassuring that your reproductive track is in reasonably good order.

How Is a Sample Collected?

Prior to semen analysis, ejaculation should be avoided for two to three days. The specimen is best analysed within an hour or two of collection for accurate results. It is recommended that up to three separate samples are taken over a six to eight week period to ensure good quality testing and to eliminate lab errors.

Normal Results

Normally, seminal fluid is clear to milky-white in colour, thick and sticky (viscous) in consistency, has a pH (acidity) level between 7.8 and 8.0, and contains few or no white blood cells (leucocytes). A healthy semen sample should contain at least twenty million sperm per ml of semen; have at least 15 per cent normally shaped sperm; and have more than 50 per cent of sperm with forward movement, or 25 per cent with rapid movement within 1 hour of ejaculation. Good sperm motility is the single most important measure of semen quality and can compensate for men with low sperm counts.

Although semen analysis can often suggest male infertility, the results may not identify the cause of the condition. Additionally, some men with low sperm counts are able to reproduce (i.e. are fertile). In many cases, abnormal semen analysis results require additional testing.

Other Tests for Fertility

Other tests that may be carried out to look at male fertility include analysis of urine to rule out infection. A full screen may be indicated to check for sexually transmitted infections; this would include penile swabs. Blood tests may look at your thyroid, liver and kidney functions, and check your iron and white cell count, as well as blood sugar levels to rule out diabetes. Hormone tests may include serum testosterone and others such as LH and FSH (hormones made by the pituitary gland in the brain: LH stimulates the testes to produce testosterone and FSH stimulates the production of sperm).

Your weight, body mass index and abdominal circumference can be checked to rule out obesity. More specialised tests may include analysis of your chromosomes and checking the immune system, particularly looking for anti-sperm antibodies that may target and attack your own sperm.

Treatment of Infertility

There are a variety of ways to treat infertility, which ultimately depend on the underlying cause. It may involve simple education and counselling, medicines to treat infections, surgery or, in some cases, highly specialised procedures such as in vitro fertilisation.

Lifestyle changes may also help alleviate infertility, such as reducing stress, dietary modification, stopping the use of drugs or alcohol, or reducing the temperature around the testes.

Other specialised treatment will depend on the underlying cause. Chronic medical illnesses, such as cirrhosis, kidney failure, sickle-cell disease or haemochromatosis, may respond to proper treatment of the underlying condition. Male infertility can be treated successfully in many cases.

Drug Therapies

Drug therapy for male infertility includes medications to improve sperm production, treat hormonal dysfunction, cure infections that compromise sperm, and fight anti-sperm antibodies. Hormone therapy may be effective in cases of testosterone deficiency. Antibiotics may be used to treat infections of the urinary tract, testes and prostate, as well as STIs that can impair fertility.

Assisted Reproduction Therapy

These are specialised procedures, such as artificial insemination, whereby the woman is injected with carefully prepared sperm from the husband, partner or a donor.

IVF or in vitro fertilisation was originally devised as a means of helping infertile women who had blocked tubes. However, this technique has now been expanded to help men with fertility issues. Human ova can be fertilised using this technique for some men with low sperm counts.

GIFT (gamete intrafallopian transfer) is a technique in which eggs or ova are retrieved in a manner similar to IVF but here the sperm are mixed together with the egg and both are injected directly into the fallopian tube for fertilisation to occur. This can be a successful treatment option for some men who are infertile.

How Can I Improve My Fertility?

It is generally accepted that the sperm count of men has been declining in recent years. There may be many varied reasons for this. Breakdown products of the female contraceptive pill in recycled drinking water have been suggested as a possible factor. Other environmental, dietary and lifestyle changes may interfere with men's sperm production. Therefore improving your diet and making healthy lifestyle choices can help your own fertility and reproductive health.

If you smoke, stop. Amongst many other adverse health effects, cigarette smoke lowers both sperm count and its ability to move.

Consuming excess amounts of alcohol reduces both the quantity and quality of sperm, so keep within recommended limits of no more than 21 units per week. Recreational drugs such as cannabis can also be associated with sluggish and unusually shaped sperm.

Being physically active and fit is also good for your fertility. Aim for at least 30 minutes of exercise a day and more if possible.

Carrying excess body fat can potentially affect your hormones so keep your belly in shape, in other words less than 37 inches in girth. Generally your body mass index should be less than 25 unless you are very muscular.

Because infertility is sometimes caused by sexually transmitted infections, practising safer sex behaviours may minimise the risk of future infertility. Gonorrhoea and chlamydia are the two most frequent causes of STI-related infertility. STIs are often asymptomatic so using a condom is essential.

Mumps immunisation has been well demonstrated to prevent mumps and its male complication, orchitis. Immunisation with the MMR vaccine prevents mumps-related sterility.

Nutrition

A healthy diet is essential for optimal health and the reproductive system is no exception. In order for your body to function properly, a well-balanced diet, including plenty of vitamins and minerals, is necessary. Nutritional deficiencies can impair hormone function, inhibit sperm production and contribute to the production of abnormal sperm.

The general rules are to eat a natural diet with foods that focus on fresh fruit and vegetables, wholegrains, fish, poultry, beans, legumes, nuts and seeds. Eat plenty of seeds, particularly pumpkin seeds, which are naturally high in zinc and essential fatty acids, both of which are vital to the healthy functioning of the male reproductive system. Foods that are rich in zinc, such as wholegrain cereals and selenium, which is found in cereals grown in selenium-rich soil as well as in Brazil nuts and mushrooms, are also important. Drink plenty of water each day.

Eliminate processed foods, junk food and sugars, and avoid stodgy carbohydrates such as breads and cakes made with white flour. Avoid hydrogenated oils (trans-fats) and minimise your saturated fat intake; use extra virgin olive oil instead. Minimise your caffeine intake and keep your alcohol intake within safe limits.

What About Supplements?

The following supplements have been suggested to be good for the male reproductive tract. Make sure you do not exceed the daily recommended limits. Remember it is always preferable to get vitamins and minerals naturally through dietary sources rather than taking them in pill form. A multivitamin is not a substitute for a bad diet. With those provisos in mind, the following supplements may help:

- Folic acid (400mcg/day) – women are told to take folic acid to help prevent serious birth defects like spina bifida, and men also need folic acid to maintain sperm quality.
- The B vitamins, especially Vitamins B_6 and B_{12}, are essential for good reproductive health.

- Vitamin C (1,000mg/day) can help prevent sperm from clumping together.
- Zinc (15–30mg/day) – low levels of zinc can also affect sperm count and motility.
- Selenium (55–100mcg/day), which is an antioxidant that helps protect the body from free radicals, can help increase sperm count and motility in men with a low sperm count.
- Vitamin E (15mg/day) has been found to aid in conception.

Herbal Medicine

Herbal remedies have been used to treat male fertility. It is important to let your doctor know if you are taking any over-the-counter supplements, including herbs, as there may be potential side effects and also potential interactions with prescribed medication. The following herbs are sometimes taken by men to help their fertility:

- Ginseng – known as a male tonic (an agent that improves general health)
- Saw palmetto (*Serenoa repens*) – used for overall male reproductive health

When to Contact Your Doctor

As couples nowadays often spend time focusing on contraception and avoiding unplanned pregnancy, there can be an assumption that pregnancy should follow as soon as a couple start 'trying'. Nothing could be further from the truth. Indeed, we generally only recommend tests or investigations if a couple have been trying for a year with no results. It is important for the couple to recognise and discuss the emotional impact that infertility has on them as individuals and as a couple, and to seek medical help and advice from their doctor. For a man there can be the added self-esteem issues of not feeling like a 'real man'. Professional counselling can be invaluable in helping to deal with these issues.

A cause can be determined for the majority of infertile couples and appropriate therapy can help many couples achieve their desired outcome.

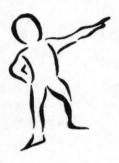

Key Points

- Male fertility is a complex process and can a sensitive issue for Irish men and their partners.
- Male infertility is a common cause of the infertility experienced by up to one in every six couples.
- Male infertility can be caused by many different factors, including lifestyle, hormonal and genetic factors, and infection.
- In many cases male fertility problems can be treated.
- A healthy lifestyle can help with your fertility.

11

Watch What You Catch!
Close the Door on Sexually
Transmitted Infections

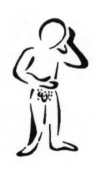 Sexually transmitted infections (STIs) are on the rise in Irish men. In the last few years, Ireland has fallen victim to a silent epidemic of sexually transmitted infections. One of the consequences of the Celtic Tiger has been the explosion in relatively cheap foreign travel opportunities. However, in some cases, men are bringing back much more than their suntan and duty-free. Despite all the information available about the importance of safe sex, more men than ever are becoming infected with STIs. Risk-taking behaviour is described as being a naturally male thing, particularly for young men. Many men continue to play Russian roulette with their sexual health.

What Are STIs?

Sexually transmitted infections (STIs) are diseases or infections that are transmitted by oral, anal or vaginal sexual intercourse. They are caused by bacteria, viruses and other organisms that can be present in blood, semen, bodily fluids or the pubic area of an infected person.

The Price We Pay

Sexually transmitted infections are one of the ways in which we pay for being irresponsible when we are sexually active. This price, for many men, can be a heavy one.

HIV infection is undoubtedly the most serious of all STIs, as it remains incurable. HIV can be fatal or at best lead to chronic lifelong illness requiring daily medication. Hepatitis B and C infections can cause chronic liver disease or liver cancer. Syphilis can actually lead to insanity if left untreated. Herpes, once caught, is a friend for life. Other infections like chlamydia can damage the reproductive organs in women, leading to long-term infertility, which can have devastating consequences for couples trying to conceive a baby. Other STIs may not pose the same degree of threat to personal health, but that does not mean that they cannot cause both pain and embarrassment, not to mention long-term health problems.

Unprotected sex with a variety of partners will inevitably lead to a sexually transmitted infection at some stage. These encounters often occur within the context of too much alcohol or other drugs, when one's guard is down. Alcohol or illicit drugs will lower inhibitions and cloud one's ability to judge safe sexual activity from irresponsible sex.

STIs tend to hunt in packs, so if you get one STI then you are more likely to have another. The fact that STI rates continue to rocket in Ireland amongst Irish men indicates either a lack of knowledge about the risks or a 'could not happen to me' attitude of denial. The more irresponsibly one behaves sexually, the greater the chance of becoming infected. Remember, sleeping with a new partner is like sleeping with everyone they have ever slept with.

It is not possible to judge whether a person is infected with an STI by sight – it requires medical testing, which is why it is safest to take precautions when having sex. Your lover may not even know themselves if they have an infection. Sometimes it can be difficult to detect an STI infection. Whenever an obvious symptom does develop you should visit your GP or local STI clinic.

Symptoms and Signs of an STI

If you are sexually active and notice any of the following symptoms, you should make an appointment to see your doctor as soon as possible:

- Pain or a burning sensation while urinating
- Pain during intercourse
- Itching or irritation in the genital area
- Any unusual discharge from your penis
- Pain or discomfort in the genital area
- A rash on the skin or genitals
- Soft, cauliflower-like bumps or blisters on genital areas
- Swollen glands, with or without sore throat and fever
- Red bumps that turn into painful blisters or sores on the penis, buttocks or thighs
- Severe fatigue, aches and pains, nausea and vomiting, loss of appetite, darkening of urine, abdominal tenderness, or yellowing of the skin and whites of the eyes (called jaundice)
- Unexplained weight loss, flu-like symptoms, persistent fevers, night sweats, headaches
- Blood in your urine or faeces

Remember, not all STIs have symptoms. Men often have no symptoms. Because of this fewer men seek treatment, and many are carriers without even knowing it. People who have no symptoms can still have an STI and can spread it to others.

Getting Tested

If you have symptoms that suggest an STI or if you have had unprotected sex, do not delay to get yourself checked out. This can be done confidentially by your own family doctor, or alternatively you can go to an STI clinic.

The sooner an STI is diagnosed and treated, the greater the chance of it being properly treated without complications. It is also important to alert your partner, as they need to be examined and treated if necessary. Diagnosis usually involves analysis of swabs taken from any unusual sores or discharge. In some cases a urine or blood test is also required. Do not be embarrassed; it is worse to live in ignorance than to put your own long-term health and that of your partner at risk.

STIs in Men – The Not So Good, the Bad and the Downright Ugly

- Genital warts
- Crabs (pubic lice)
- Chlamydia
- Gonorrhoea
- Syphilis
- Genital herpes
- Hepatitis B and C
- HIV/AIDS

Genital Warts

This is the most common STI in Ireland. Genital warts are caused by the human papillomavirus (HPV), which is a cousin of the virus that causes hand warts. Genital warts are highly contagious and can have a very long incubation period, meaning they may not appear for up to a year after exposure. Genital warts in themselves are not a serious infection in men but they may indicate the presence of other STIs, which must be screened for and appropriately treated.

Infection with the human papillomavirus is the leading cause of cervical cancer in women. Therefore wearing a condom can not only protect you against acquiring sexually transmitted infections but can also potentially protect your partner against cervical cancer.

What Do Genital Warts Look Like?

Genital warts are small cauliflower-shaped growths usually seen on the penis. Warts can also appear on the scrotum or around the anus and may spread around the anus without you having had anal sex. Sometimes the warts can be seen around and in the mouth and throat of those who have had oral sex with an infected person.

What Is the Treatment for Genital Warts?

Genital warts are treated with lotions or creams prescribed by your doctor. Sometimes the warts can be frozen off with liquid nitrogen in a process known as cryotherapy. It is probable that you may require more than one type of treatment before the warts go. Unfortunately, like most viruses, there is no treatment that will get rid of the virus itself. The genital warts can be treated; however, they may reappear at a later stage.

Crabs (Pubic Lice)

Pubic lice or 'crabs' are crab-shaped insects that can take up residence in the pubic hair. Crabs like the warm moist areas of our bodies so can also be found in the armpits, in facial hair and sometimes even in eyelashes. The adult lice feed on human blood and lay their eggs, or nits, on the hair shafts close to the skin.

You get crabs by direct close physical contact with someone who already has them. They can occasionally be caught from the towels, bed sheets or clothes of an infested person. The lice can only survive for between 24 and 48 hours away from the human body.

Symptoms of Pubic Lice

Pubic lice can cause severe itch in the genital area. The lice may be seen crawling around on the pubic area. The eggs of the lice may be seen as black specks on pubic hair. After the eggs hatch a baby louse, called a nymph, emerges. They are smaller versions of the adults they become after seven days. Adult crabs are visible to the naked eye but because of their gray, white or brown colour are difficult to see as they can easily blend in with their surroundings. You may see faint blue spots where they have bitten you.

Treatment of Pubic Lice

There are a number of topical treatments available either from your pharmacy or on prescription from your doctor. It is important to follow the instructions carefully. This includes all appropriate measures to prevent re-infection such as:

- Washing all your sheets, towels and clothes
- Putting other pieces of clothing into a plastic bag for thirty days, in which time all the lice will die
- Informing your sexual partner so they are also treated

- Avoiding intimate contact until treatment has been completed
- Cleaning your bathroom and shower with bathroom cleaner or bleach

Chlamydia

Chlamydia (pronounced klam-id-e-a) is a sexually transmitted infection that is easy to pass on during unprotected sexual contact through vaginal, anal or oral sex. Chlamydia infection is common among sexually active men. It often has no symptoms and is therefore known as a silent infection.

Signs and Symptoms of Chlamydia

Men with chlamydia can have a penile discharge. Chlamydia can cause pain and discomfort while urinating. It can also cause you to urinate more often and you can have a burning and itching sensation around the opening of the penis. Sometimes it can cause swelling of the lining of the testicles, which is known as epididymitis. It can also lead to inflammation of the prostate gland, known as prostatitis. Untreated chlamydia can lead to eye problems and a form of arthritis known as Reiter's syndrome.

Unfortunately chlamydia can be an even more serious infection for women, causing pelvic inflammatory disease, ectopic pregnancy and sometimes infertility.

Testing For and Treating Chlamydia

Chlamydia is diagnosed in men by either a urine test or by taking a swab from the penis. It is easily treated with antibiotics. It is important if you have chlamydia that you abstain from sexual intercourse until you and your sexual partner have completed treatment. If you don't, you will simply get re-infected. A test to ensure you are cured can be carried out several weeks after treatment but is generally not necessary. Unfortunately, there are many men out there who don't know they have chlamydia, with the result that they are infecting and sometimes re-infecting their female partners.

Gonorrhoea

Gonorrhoea is a bacterial infection commonly known as 'the clap'. Gonorrhoea is caused by bacteria called *Neisseria gonorrhoeae*, which love the warm, moist linings of the mouth, rectum, vagina and urethra. Gonorrhoea can be successfully treated with antibiotics. There are about 200 million cases of gonorrhoea worldwide.

Symptoms of Gonorrhoea in Men

Symptoms can develop up to a month after exposure and include discomfort in the penis, a discharge from the tip of the penis, and pain or a burning sensation when urinating. This discharge is often greenish or yellow in colour. Other symptoms may include painful testicular swelling or inflammation of the prostate gland. About one in ten infected men will not have any symptoms of gonorrhoea.

Gonorrhoea infection following anal sex can result in soreness and itching with a possible anal discharge. Sometimes this is accompanied by severe pain, especially when defaecating. On the other hand, there may be no symptoms except a moist feeling in the rectum. The infection is passed on during subsequent anal intercourse.

Gonorrhoea infection of the mouth can result in inflammation of the throat.

Testing For and Treating Gonorrhoea

In order to test for gonorrhoea, swabs are taken from the urethra and throat, and a rectal swab is also taken if applicable, and these are examined under the microscope.

Treatment for gonorrhoea with antibiotics is usually successful. A new drug-resistant strain of gonorrhoea, now found in many countries, can make treatment more difficult. A second test is needed following treatment to confirm that the infection has gone. Untreated gonorrhoea can lead to a form of arthritis. It is also important that your partner is tested and appropriately treated because, in women, untreated gonorrhoea can lead to infertility.

Syphilis

Syphilis is a sexually transmitted disease that has been around since at least the sixteenth century. It is caused by bacteria called *Treponema pallidum*, which like the warm moist linings of the genital passages, rectum and mouth, but die quickly outside the body. Syphilis is commonly known as 'the pox' and it has been called 'the great mimic' because it can produce so many different symptoms in the body.

Symptoms of Syphilis

Syphilis often begins with a crusty sore on the penis. Swelling of the glands in the groin may occur. The sore heals after a few weeks without treatment. However the syphilis bug has not gone away and it continues to spread throughout the body. After several weeks you may start to feel unwell, with flu-like symptoms, swollen glands and a rash. These symptoms can last for several months.

Treatments for Syphilis

The main treatment for syphilis is antibiotics, usually penicillin, which can completely cure it. Without treatment, syphilis can hide in the body for many years before reappearing to potentially cause blindness, dementia, insanity or death from a ruptured aneurysm.

Genital Herpes

Genital herpes is caused by the herpes simplex virus type 2 (HSV-2). This is related to the herpes simplex virus type 1, which causes cold sores on the mouth or lips. Symptoms are tiny blisters on the penis, sometimes with a temperature, tiredness and swollen glands in the groin region. This tends to occur within about a week of exposure to the herpes virus. Without treatment, genital herpes tends to settle down after a week or so. However the infection can reoccur at any time, even without further sexual exposure. Antiviral medication can speed recovery from outbreaks of herpes, but it is not curable.

Hepatitis

The hepatitis A virus is not an STI. However the hepatitis B and C viruses can be spread through sexual contact or by the exchange of bodily fluids, such as blood, saliva or urine, with an infected person. Symptoms include tiredness, jaundice and flu-like aches and pains.

These viruses can cause serious liver inflammation, which may lead to liver damage, liver failure and liver cancer. Infection is confirmed by means of a blood test. There is an excellent vaccine to protect against hepatitis B, which can be given to people at risk of infection. Hepatitis C can be treated with certain antiviral agents. Unfortunately there is no vaccine available to protect against hepatitis C.

HIV and AIDS

Since it was first identified about twenty-seven years ago, HIV has become a global catastrophe, infecting millions of people annually. HIV is an extremely deadly virus because it affects our natural immune system. It destroys the white blood cells that are needed to fight infection. By destroying the body's own immune system the floodgates to infection are opened. Therefore the system becomes overrun with bacterial, fungal and viral infections. Fortunately, medical breakthroughs in recent years have led to the development of new antiviral medicine: anti-HIV drug 'cocktails'. These allow many people to survive HIV/AIDS and live active lives. To benefit most from these antiviral drugs, HIV/AIDS must be diagnosed early.

If you have had unprotected exposure to the HIV virus, make sure to get yourself tested. Blood tests can accurately diagnose HIV. However, there is a recognised window period, meaning that it may take some time – at least three months and sometimes longer – after unprotected exposure to HIV before the test may show up positive in your blood.

Signs and Symptoms of HIV/AIDS

Early signs of HIV/AIDS infection can include flu-like symptoms, unexplained rashes, fungal infections in the throat, swollen glands and unusual tiredness. These symptoms and signs are similar to many different flu-like or viral infections and diseases. The person appears to recover, usually between a week and a month later. Often, however, early infection with HIV/AIDS has no symptoms.

Later signs and symptoms of HIV/AIDS can include rapid weight loss, dry cough, fevers or night sweats, fatigue, swollen lymph glands in the armpits, groin or neck, recurrent infections such as chest infections, pneumonia or *candida* infections (thrush) in the mouth, memory loss and depression. At this stage the person is said to have progressed from having a HIV infection to having full-blown AIDS. As the disease progresses and the immune system is weakened further, cancers and other life-threatening infections can occur.

Many people who carry the HIV virus don't know they are infected; that's why being tested is so important. If you are sexually active with more than one partner – or have any reason to think you might have been exposed to HIV in the past – go to your doctor and discuss whether you should be screened or not.

Can STIs Be Prevented?

Yes, in fact STIs are easily prevented. The only foolproof way is to avoid sex. The next best way to prevent an STI is simply to have sex with an uninfected partner in the context of a monogamous, faithful relationship. The third way is to always practise safe sex. Using condoms that prevent the sharing of body fluids cuts down on the likelihood of cross-infection, but occasionally they do fail during use. However, they are still highly effective at preventing the spread of STIs.

There is no doubt that there is a big knowledge deficit among men when it comes to men's sexual health issues, as with other health-related areas. The challenge is to provide information and education about sexually transmitted infections so that men can make informed choices. It is also important that equal emphasis is put on alcohol and drug awareness as unplanned sexual encounters often occur in the context of alcohol and/or drug use.

A useful acronym for prevention is 'ABC':

- **A**bstinence
- **B**e faithful
- Use a **C**ondom

Condoms

Because the pill is taken by many women to prevent pregnancy, men may feel they are off the hook when it comes to taking responsibility for sexual health issues. If avoiding pregnancy is your aim then the birth control pill can be quite effective, though not 100 per cent so. However, the pill is of no use whatsoever in blocking the transmission of an STI. Only condoms have been demonstrated to prevent the spread of STIs during sexual contact. However, it seems that even the fear of catching AIDS has not stopped people from having unsafe sex. Like most things in life, using a condom is simple once you know how. Condoms help prevent the spread of sexually transmitted infections and can also be an effective form of family planning.

Some men are allergic to latex products, including condoms. Most condoms are made of latex so men with a latex allergy should consider using a natural membrane, but these are less effective in terms of preventing pregnancy, so additional precautions should be taken.

Some of the Reasons for Condom Failure

- Condoms breaking during sex – condoms can sometimes break, especially with vigorous sexual activity.
- Defective condoms – the kitemark standard shows that the manufacturer tests their products to a high standard. Tests on condoms include water volume and air burst tests, but not a friction test.
- Not using appropriate lubricant – if you are using a lubricant make sure it is water- or silicone-based, such as glycerin or lubricating jellies (which can be purchased at any pharmacy). NEVER use oil-based lubricants such as petroleum jelly, cold cream, hand lotion or baby oil with a condom as they will weaken the condom and can cause it to disintegrate.
- Using an expired condom – take the expiry date seriously, because condoms can lose their elasticity and become defective. After that date, the condom may not provide the protection you need to avoid pregnancy or infection.
- Re-using condoms – remember always use a new condom each time you have sex. Never re-use a condom and always dispose of it after use.

If you do not protect yourself each time you have sex then you risk getting and passing on a sexually transmitted infection.

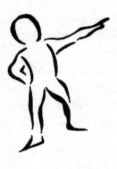

Key Points

- Sexually transmitted infections are on the increase.
- These infections may have no symptoms.
- There can be serious long-term effects.
- Be responsible and practise safe sex.
- Wear a condom.
- Remember ABC – **A**bstinence; **B**e faithful; use a **C**ondom.

12

Know Your Balls

As men we normally have two balls, or testes, which are located in a pouch or sac of skin, called the scrotum, underneath our penis. They are easy to feel and check, yet many men never do so. This is a pity because testicular cancer is common in young men and is also easily curable if caught early. So, for the sake of your health, you should know your balls. Of course, many simple testicular problems have nothing to do with cancer at all and some of the more important and common conditions are described in this chapter.

Get to Know Your Testes (Testicles)

The testicles are the male sex glands and are part of the male reproductive system. In adult men, each one is normally somewhat smaller than a golf ball. The spermatic cord is like a flexible tube that goes from each testis to the lower abdomen. The spermatic cord contains the blood vessels that take blood to and from the testis, and the vas deferens which take sperm from the testis to the penis.

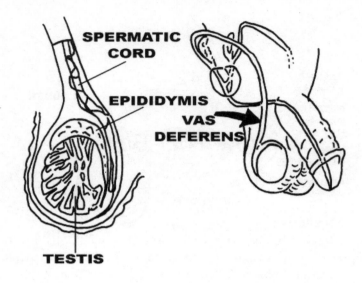

What Do The Testicles Do?

Firstly, they make the male hormone testosterone. This hormone is responsible for the development of the reproductive organs and other male characteristics, such as body and facial hair, deep voice and broad shoulders. Secondly, they produce and store sperm, which carry the genetic code to create a baby. Sperm cells are carried from the testicles through small tubes called the vas deferens to the seminal vesicles. Fluid from the vesicles and from the prostate gland is added. During ejaculation (orgasm), this fluid, now called semen, travels through a tube (the urethra) in the centre of the penis and out of the body.

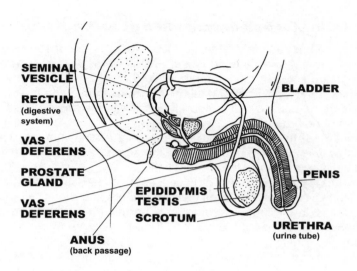

SEMINAL VESICLE

RECTUM (digestive system)

VAS DEFERENS

PROSTATE GLAND

VAS DEFERENS

ANUS (back passage)

EPIDIDYMIS
TESTIS

SCROTUM

BLADDER

PENIS

URETHRA (urine tube)

Self-Examination

By examining yourself regularly, you will be more confident about your own body and in a better position to notice any changes in a previously normal testicle. If you notice any change in the size of a testis, or any abnormal lumps, swellings or tender spots, then you should see your doctor. Doctors are used to examining testes and will be able to advise if the abnormality is serious or not.

It is important to remember that most abnormalities are not cancer. However, cancer of the testes is the most common cancer in young men in Ireland and affects about one in every 500 men between the ages of 15 and 50. If it is caught early, it can almost always be easily treated and cured. Therefore, it is important to practise regular testicular self-examination so that you get to know how your testes normally feel. This allows any changes to be more easily detected.

Testicular Self-Examination (TSE) Procedure

- Practise this regularly, at least once a month. The best time for testicular self-examination is just after a warm bath or shower, when the scrotal tissue is more relaxed.
- While standing in front of a mirror, place the thumbs on the front side of the testicle and support it with the index and middle fingers of both hands.
- Gently roll the testicle between the fingers and thumbs. The testes can move around a little in the scrotum, but cannot usually move enough to twist round fully.
- Feel for lumps, hardness or thickness. Compare the feelings in each testicle. Normal testes feel like smooth and slightly spongy balls inside the baggy scrotum. It is normal for one testis to be slightly bigger than the other, and for one to hang slightly lower than the other.
- You can normally feel the spermatic cord through the skin of the scrotum just above the testis. It feels like a thick piece of string.
- If you find any swelling, lump, unusual tenderness or other abnormality, see your doctor as soon as possible.

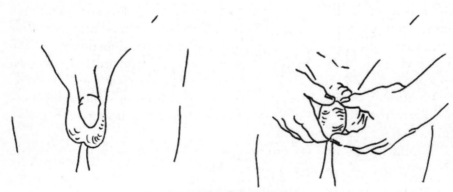

SELF-EXAMINATION

What Is Epididymo-Orchitis?

Orchitis means inflammation of a testis (testicle). Epididymitis means inflammation of the epididymis (the structure next to the testis that is involved in making sperm). Because the testes and epididymis lie so close together in the scrotum, it is often difficult to know whether either or both are inflamed.

Most cases are due to an infection:

- Urinary tract infection – bugs that cause urinary tract infection can spread into the testes and epididymis, causing epididymo-orchitis.
- Sexually transmitted infections – in young men this is the most common cause. It is most commonly seen with chlamydia and gonorrhoea infections.
- Mumps – this used to be a common cause but is now uncommon thanks to the MMR vaccine. Mumps can cause epididymo-orchitis in about one in every five cases.
- Uncommon causes include other types of infections from other parts of the body that can, rarely, travel in the blood to the testes.

Symptoms come on over a day or so and include a swollen, tender and red scrotum. It may feel warm to touch as well as sore. You may have a temperature and generally feel unwell. There may be other symptoms, such as burning when passing urine, depending on the underlying cause. If a urinary tract or sexually transmitted infection appears to be the cause then a urine test or penile swabs will be done.

Treatment usually involves a course of antibiotics and symptoms normally resolve over a week or so. Supporting underwear sometimes helps to ease the pain.

Complications are uncommon and a full recovery is the norm. However possible complications include:

- Reduced fertility in the affected testis

- An abscess that may form in the scrotum and may need surgical treatment
- Rarely, damage to the testes – resulting in gangrene of the testes requiring surgical removal

Hydrocele

A hydrocele is a collection of fluid in the scrotum next to a testis. A hydrocele feels smooth, like a small fluid-filled balloon inside the scrotum. It usually occurs on one side, but sometimes a hydrocele forms over both testes. They vary greatly in size. Hydroceles usually have no symptoms unless they get large, in which case they may cause some discomfort.

Most hydroceles occur in older men and usually there is no underlying cause. Sometimes it may occur as a result of an infection, injury or tumour of a testis. Your doctor can diagnose a hydrocele by shining a light against the scrotal skin: a hydrocele will cause the scrotum to light up like a lantern. Sometimes an ultrasound scan of the testes is done to check the testes to make sure there is no underlying cause of the hydrocele.

Treatment options for a hydrocele include draining the fluid and repairing the hydrocele with a surgical procedure. Watchful waiting (no active treatment) can be a very reasonable option too, especially in older men. If there is an underlying problem with the testis this will need to be treated as well.

Varicoceles

A varicocele (pronounced var-ih-ko-seal) is like a swollen or varicose vein in your scrotal sac. It has been described medically as like feeling a mass of quivering worms. The majority of varicoceles are found on the left side of the scrotum. Varicoceles are common and can affect about one in every seven young men. Most of the time a varicocele does not mean any underlying serious condition, but occasionally it can be due to other problems in the abdomen, such as a kidney tumour.

What Are the Symptoms?

Varicoceles are usually painless and have no symptoms. Some men may notice a 'dragging' feeling or slight discomfort from their varicocele. This may only occur at the end of the day, especially if you were on your feet all day.

Are Varicoceles Serious?

They are usually harmless. There is a higher rate of infertility in men with a varicocele compared to those who do not have one. This may be due to the increased temperature in the testes caused by the swollen veins. The testis on the side of the varicocele can become smaller, or not develop as much as the other side. This may contribute to infertility too. If you are infertile and you have a varicocele, your specialist will be able to advise on current research related to this issue. Sometimes, if they are large, they can be treated surgically.

Torsion of the Testis

Torsion of the testis is a condition that requires an emergency operation. It occurs when a testis twists around in the scrotum. In some people the testes can move around in the scrotum more than usual. If a testis twists round, the blood supply to the testis is blocked in the twisted spermatic cord. The effect of this is that the testis, with its blood supply cut off, becomes damaged and will 'die' unless the blood flow is quickly restored.

Torsion is most common in teenage boys, shortly after puberty, and it is uncommon in men over the age of 25.

TORSION OF TESTIS

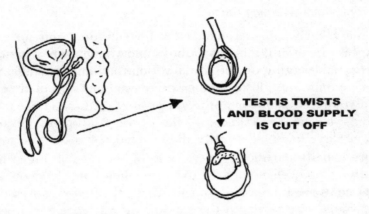

TESTIS TWISTS AND BLOOD SUPPLY IS CUT OFF

What Are the Symptoms of Torsion of the Testis?

The main symptom of torsion is severe pain in the testicle. Sometimes pain is also felt in the belly area due to the nerve supply to the testes. The pain tends to come on quite quickly and becomes severe over a few hours. The affected testis soon becomes swollen, red and very sore to touch.

What Is the Treatment for Torsion of the Testis?

Torsion of the testis is an emergency because if the blood supply to the testis is cut off for more than about 6 hours, permanent damage to the testis is likely to result. An emergency operation is usually done to untwist the testis and spermatic cord and 'fix' the testis in position so that torsion can't happen again. There is an increased chance of torsion occurring in the other testis at a later date so that testis is also fixed at the same time to prevent this from happening.

The operation ideally should be within a few hours of the symptoms starting in order to maximize the chance of saving the testis. Otherwise, the testis may have to be removed.

Partial Torsion and Warning Pains

Sometimes sharp pains, which last a few minutes and go just as quickly, can occur in the testes of boys and young men. This can be due to partial twisting of the testis, which then untwists again with relief of symptoms. This can be an early warning sign of a possible torsion later on. It is important to get prompt medical advice if these symptoms occur. Sometimes if these warning pains occur, an operation is recommended to fix the affected testis so as to prevent full-blown torsion later on.

Blood In the Semen

The presence of blood in the ejaculate is called haematospermia (pronounced hem-at-o-sperm-e-a). This is usually a harmless symptom; however, it can cause major worry and anxiety for an affected man. Usually there is no underlying medical cause and detailed investigations are not needed. Less commonly, it may be associated with abnormalities of the urinary tract, including kidney and prostate problems, and occasionally is associated with other more generalised illnesses, such as cirrhosis of the liver or parasitic infections. Men aged over 40 with persistent haematospermia may need to be referred to a urologist, especially if they have other symptoms or abnormal findings on examination.

Hernia

The muscle wall of the stomach area normally forms a good protective barrier to the intestines that lie underneath it. If this muscle wall weakens in an area then the intestines can bulge through. This is called a hernia. Hernias occur most commonly in the groin area as this is usually the weakest point of the abdominal muscle wall. Sometimes hernias can be seen elsewhere, such as at the site of an old operation scar or near the belly button. Occasionally, particularly in obese individuals, a hernia occurs in the centre of the abdominal wall where the muscle layers join together. Over time hernias can increase in size and sometimes hernias in the groin area can track all the way down into the scrotum.

The main symptom is a bulge or lump felt under the skin. A hernia may be first noticed after a strain, for example, lifting a heavy object or coughing. This lump can usually be pushed back at first. Hernias may cause a sense of discomfort but they are not usually painful.

Hernias can be successfully treated by a small operation, which can normally be done as a day case procedure. A stitch or mesh is put into the weakened muscle area to strengthen it. It is important not to do any heavy lifting for several weeks after this procedure to minimise the chance of recurrence.

Treatment to fix a hernia is normally advised because, if untreated, it may become bigger with time. There is also a small chance that a hernia might strangulate. This is where the bowel bulging through the gap in the muscle twists, cutting off its blood supply. This can cause severe pain and requires an emergency operation to fix it. It is not unlike torsion of the testis. Fortunately, strangulation of a hernia is uncommon but it is a good reason to have your hernia fixed routinely.

Peyronie's Disease of the Penis

Peyronie's disease is a condition of the penis where firm rope-like or fibrous plaques form in the soft spongy tissue of the penis. These plaques don't stretch so that, when the man develops an erection, the penis tends to bend. Sometimes this bend can become so severe that sexual intercourse becomes impossible. Peyronie's disease is not linked to either infection or cancer of the penis.

Who Can Get Peyronie's Disease?

Any man can develop Peyronie's disease. It usually occurs in men aged over 40, but can be seen in younger men.

What Are the Causes and Symptoms?

The exact cause is not yet fully understood. In some men there may be a family history of this condition. Many men who get Peyronie's disease also have diabetes or heart disease. Some men who get Peyronie's disease also have Dupuytren's contracture, which is a similar fibrotic condition found in the tendons in the palm of the hand that causes a progressive bending, usually of the fourth finger. The main symptoms of Peyronie's disease are:

- Penile pain on erection
- A thickening in the shaft of the penis
- A curvature of the erect penis
- Sometimes erectile dysfunction (ED or impotence) as well

The first symptom tends to be penile pain and discomfort, which occurs with an erection as the plaque is stretched. This pain with an erection usually goes within a few months. The next thing the affected man notices is a thickened feeling or lump (plaque) in the shaft of his penis. After this he may notice that the penis tends to become more curved when erect. This can make sexual intercourse more difficult and uncomfortable and it may eventually become impossible. Erectile dysfunction is commonly seen in men with Peyronie's disease.

How Is Peyronie's Disease Treated?

Fortunately, many men with Peyronie's disease have a mild form of the condition, which doesn't interfere with sexual intercourse. These men need no treatment. For men with more severe forms of the condition, several treatment options can be tried, including injections into the penile plaques or surgery to try to straighten the penis. Unfortunately there is no guarantee of success, as the underlying cause of Peyronie's disease remains unknown.

What Is a Vasectomy?

A vasectomy is a simple and highly effective method of contraception. It is sometimes known as male sterilisation. A vasectomy is a procedure that involves cutting the two tubes leading away from the testes, called the vas deferens, so that sperm can no longer get into the semen. A vasectomy is usually considered to be a permanent form of contraception, although in some cases the procedure can be reversed, if necessary (but with difficulty).

A vasectomy works by preventing sperm from reaching the semen that is ejaculated from the man's penis during sex. It is a quick and usually painless surgical procedure, which is carried out under local anaesthetic. This means that, in most cases, you will be able to return home within an hour or so of your procedure.

What Are the Risks of a Vasectomy?

The risk of side effects or complications after a vasectomy is low and these are usually minor; they may include some bleeding or bruising at the scrotum. Mild infection is uncommon. Less commonly, a swelling called a sperm granuloma may occur due to an inflammatory reaction to sperm released into the bloodstream or tissue during the procedure. Much rarer is when the ends of the vas deferens may reconnect with one another, which could result in your partner getting pregnant.

There is currently no evidence of any increased risks of prostate cancer or other long-term health complications. However, these matters are the subject of ongoing research.

A vasectomy shouldn't affect your sex drive or ability to have erections or orgasm. The only difference is that the semen you ejaculate will not contain sperm. The body continues to produce sperm after the procedure, but the testicles naturally reabsorb the unneeded sperm.

Will the Vasectomy Work Right Away?

After the procedure it is generally recommended to use additional precautions until a sperm test is done after four months or so. If this is clear then sex can take place without additional precautions.

How Well Does It Work?

Vasectomy is a very effective method of permanent birth control. The figures say only about 15 out of 10,000 couples get pregnant the first year after a vasectomy. It is a permanent procedure, so, as a couple, you need to be sure that your family is complete. Remember, a vasectomy does not give any protection against sexually transmitted infections (STIs). Condoms are the most effective method of preventing STIs. To protect yourself and your partner from STIs, use a condom every time you have sex.

The Male Menopause – Fact or Fiction?

The menopause is the name given to the change that occurs in women when their ovaries (the parts of the female body that make eggs) start to shut down, causing a rapid drop in female hormone levels. The effects of this in women include symptoms like hot flushes, sweats and mood swings, as well as loss of fertility. Age-related hormone changes are very different in men than in women. Levels of the male hormone (testosterone) do start to gradually decline in men from the age of 40 onwards, but there is no rapid drop in hormone levels. So the term 'male menopause' is not an accurate description.

For the majority of ageing men, testosterone levels, while reducing, still remain in the normal range. About 20 per cent of men may experience symptoms of testosterone deficiency, which are uncommon in men under the age of 60. In recent years, testosterone replacement therapy has become available. It has received a lot of media attention as an agent to promote male strength and virility: an 'anti-ageing pill'. While there is no doubt it can be helpful for men with proven testosterone deficiency, it can have potentially serious side effects.

What Is Testosterone?

Testosterone is the male sex hormone and it has a role in:

- Keeping your bones and muscles strong
- Ensuring healthy sperm production
- Promoting the growth of facial hair

It also affects male behaviour and aggressiveness and is essential for the libido or sex drive, as well as for normal erection and sexual performance.

The changes that occur around puberty, when a boy becomes a man, are related to the effects of testosterone. These include the growth spurt of the body, deepening of the voice, development of facial hair, development of the male shape and development of the penis and testicles. If you are unfortunate enough to lose your testicles before puberty your voice will not deepen and you will always have a full head of hair.

Testosterone is made in the testicles and this is under the control of the pituitary gland, a small pea-sized gland in the brain.

What Are the Symptoms of Low Testosterone Levels?

There is huge variation here. Many men with declining testosterone levels remain symptom-free, as their testosterone levels remain in the normal range. Some men with low testosterone levels have no symptoms. The only way to diagnose testosterone deficiency with certainty is by a blood test. Symptoms vary from person to person and may overlap with symptoms of normal ageing. Testosterone deficiency, however, may be associated with the following symptoms and signs:

Physical Symptoms

- Reduced muscle size and strength
- Thinning of the bones
- Loss of height
- Osteoporosis
- Loss of body or pubic hair
- Sweating and hot flushes

Sexual Symptoms

- Reduced sex drive
- Reduction in spontaneous erections
- Infertility
- Small or shrinking testes

Psychological Symptoms

- Lack of concentration
- Loss of memory
- Lack of confidence
- Low self-esteem
- Lowering of mood
- Irritability
- Overlap with other symptoms of clinical depression

Other Symptoms

- Increase in body fat
- Less energy
- Impaired work performance
- Sleep apnoea or other sleep problems
- Mild anaemia due to a low red cell count

Many of the symptoms of testosterone deficiency can overlap with many other medical conditions. Therefore, if you feel you may be suffering from some of these symptoms, it is important to have a good chat with your family doctor, who will be able to help you decide on their likely significance.

Should I Take Testosterone Replacement Therapy (TRT)?

It all depends. This is a decision that should be taken in close consultation with your doctor, having regard to all the potential pluses and minuses (see table below). Certainly, if you have proven testosterone deficiency, there may be some benefits in terms of helping with some of the symptoms described above. Testosterone can increase muscle mass and strength, improve bone density, and boost red blood cell count. Whether it can improve libido, erectile function or sexual performance in older men remains unclear.

Advantages and Disadvantages of Testosterone Therapy

Advantages of Testosterone Therapy	Disadvantages of Testosterone Therapy
Improves muscle mass and strength	Skin effects – acne
Strengthens bones	Baldness
Thickens body hair and skin	Fluid retention
Possibly improves libido and sex drive	Sleep apnoea
More energy	Breast enlargement (gynaecomastia)
Better brain function	Breast cancer
Enhances mood – less irritability and depression	Prostate enlargement
	Prostate cancer
	Testicular shrinkage
	Reduced sperm production causing infertility
	Excess red blood cell production – causing thickening of the blood (polycythaemia), which can increase the risk of stroke

There are several types of TRT available. The most common types are a patch that is stuck onto the skin, an injection or a gel. If you are using a testosterone gel it is important to let the gel dry fully before you have contact with your partner. Otherwise she may become more muscular as well!

There is no doubt TRT can cause many potentially serious side effects. The oral tablet form of testosterone is not used as it can have serious effects both on the liver and the heart.

Testosterone can cause the prostate gland to enlarge and this enlargement of the prostate gland can put pressure on the urethra, causing prostate symptoms, such as urinating more often, difficulties with starting or stopping the stream, terminal dribbling and having to pass urine at night. Potentially much more serious is the fact that TRT can promote the growth of prostate cancer, which may already be lying dormant in the prostate gland. Therefore it is most important that you get your prostate checked out before considering going down the road of TRT. Talking to your doctor about your prostate health, combined with blood tests (PSA) and a rectal examination of the prostate, can give you a good idea of your prostate health (see Chapter 8).

Using TRT to treat low testosterone due to ageing is controversial. Despite the obvious appeal of testosterone replacement for older men, most doctors advise against it; on balance, the risks seem to outweigh the benefits. TRT has definite risks, especially in terms of prostate cancer and heart disease, and it may not improve your symptoms. TRT may also have possible long-term health risks that are not yet known.

So What About the Midlife Crisis?

There is no doubt that many men experience a bit of a midlife crisis, typically between the ages of 45 and 65. There may be many reasons for this. Mostly the physical changes that can occur in middle age, such as middle-age spread, baldness, sagging muscles and expanding waist line, are in direct conflict with media and societal images of the all-powerful male: young, athletic, muscular and sexually omnipotent. This time is often one of uncertainty for men in terms of work and career. There can be a certain loss of energy and loss of confidence, some erectile dysfunction issues and a fear of ageing. However, many of the issues and challenges at this stage of life can be successfully addressed:

- Talk to your doctor about any health concerns you may have, including any erectile dysfunction or other sexual problems.

- Remember your mental health and get help if you feel down.
- Confide in and listen to your spouse or partner.
- Focus on a healthy lifestyle by following a programme of regular exercise and a low-fat, high-fibre, vegetable- and fruit-rich diet. This can help keep you in good shape as you get older.
- Lose the beer belly – a healthy diet combined with a good exercise programme can help.
- Keep your weight down and, more importantly, the size of your belly. Keep it under 40 inches, ideally under 37 inches.
- Look at your work–life balance issues. Are you working too hard? Have you enough down time? Have you enough 'me time'?
- Keep a healthy respect for alcohol.
- Work on improving your relationships.
- Consider counselling.
- Learn to de-stress.

Make time for the 'non-urgent'; prioritise important areas of your life that can often be overlooked when you are too busy. This includes friendships, family and hobbies.

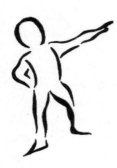

Key Points

- Know your own body and what is normal for you.
- Practise testicular self-examination regularly (see page 216).
- Be confident enough to seek help if you have any worries or concerns in this area.
- Remember your doctor is there to help you.
- Testosterone levels start to drop in many men from the age of 40.
- However, testosterone levels often stay in the normal range.

- There are many symptoms of testosterone deficiency.
- Testosterone replacement therapy has potential risks and benefits.
- A healthy lifestyle can actively combat the effects of ageing.

13

Alcohol and Drugs

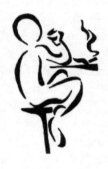

Alcohol – a Good Servant and a Bad Master

Alcohol is the most widely used and abused drug among Irish men and is a major risk factor for ill-health and premature death. Alcohol-related problems are epidemic in Irish society, as a weekend visit to an accident and emergency department in any Irish hospital will testify. Problems associated with drinking alcohol include increased numbers of accidents and injuries; increased violence; increased absenteeism from work; a risk of suffocation through choking on one's own vomit; alcohol poisoning, which is potentially fatal; and an association with many physical and mental health disorders, including depression and suicide.

There is no doubt that some men drink more when they are under stress. However, using alcohol as a means to de-stress may only give temporary relief of symptoms, followed the next day by a worsening of the stress feelings – one step forwards and two steps back!

Using alcohol as a stress buster can make you more likely to become dependent on alcohol.

There can undoubtedly be significant health and social benefits to low-dose alcohol, if drunk by the right person at the right time in the right amount. But it is very much a case of 'less is more'.

How to Calculate the Number of Units in a Drink

The system of 'units' of alcohol in drink was thought up years ago as a means of estimating the amount of alcohol in different drinks so as to work out how much alcohol someone is consuming. The strength of drink is measured as 'ABV', which means alcohol by volume.

The most accurate way to calculate the number of units in an alcoholic drink is to look at the percentage of alcohol by volume (% ABV) of a drink. This equals the number of units of alcohol in 1 litre of that drink. For example, wine with 12 per cent ABV has 12 units of alcohol in a litre of wine, so if you drink half a litre of wine (500 mls), which is four small glasses, then you have had 6 units of alcohol.

Ordinary strength beer, at 4 per cent ABV, has 4 units of alcohol in a litre, so if you drink half a litre, which is just under a pint, then you will have had 2 units of alcohol. Strong beer, at 6 per cent ABV, has 6 units in a litre, so a half litre of this equates to 3 units. So you can see that the number of units of alcohol can vary widely from beer to beer, depending on the ABV.

One unit of alcohol is about equal to:

- A half pint of ordinary strength beer (3–4% ABV) or
- A small pub measure of spirits (40% ABV) or
- A standard pub measure (50 mls) of sherry or port (20% ABV)

Calculating the number of units of alcohol in a drink isn't rocket science and certainly doesn't require a degree in maths.

How to Figure it Out

Multiply the amount of drink in millilitres by the percentage ABV and then divide the answer by 1,000. This gives the number of units in that drink. For example:

- A pint of strong beer at 8% ABV:
  1 pint (568 mls) x 8 = 4,544, divided by 1,000 = 4.5 units
- A 150 ml glass of wine at 12% ABV:
  150 mls x 12 = 1,800, divided by 1,000 = 1.8 units

It's no longer accurate to simply say a glass of wine is 1 unit of alcohol because it depends on the size of the glass as well as the strength (ABV) of the wine. Drinkers beware!

How Much Is Too Much?

The World Health Organization has recommended upper limits of alcohol intake for men at 21 units spread over the entire week. What they are saying is that consuming up to 21 units of alcohol over the full week is unlikely to harm your health. However, if you binge drink all these units in one or two days, then certainly you will harm your health. Just as you would not take a week's supply of pain killers in one day so you should not take all your weekly quota of units of alcohol in one go. In general, the more you drink above the recommended limit the more harmful alcohol is likely to be. Not only is the number of units consumed important but their timing as well. One small drink can impair your reflexes and judgement. Even a small amount of alcohol can have negative effects on some men's wellbeing. So it is important to look at the broader effects alcohol has on you and not just focus on the amount. Many men may feel they are 'grand' because they don't drink as much as their friends do. But if they look at the effects alcohol is having on them in terms of psychological or physical health, or effects on work, sport or relationships, then it may be a different story. Some men can experience negative effects from small amounts of alcohol, such as anxiety, feelings of panic and palpitations. If this is the case then clearly you shouldn't drink at all. It is important to be aware of the health issues associated with alcohol so you can make an informed decision for yourself.

Potential Health Hazards of Alcohol

There is a saying, 'less is more', and this is very true when it comes to alcohol. While a little alcohol can be good for your health, more is definitely not better. Excess alcohol can damage nearly every organ in the body and has been implicated in about sixty different diseases. This risk of damage increases when you either binge drink or consume more than 21 units per week.

The Heart

Heavy drinking increases the risk of high blood pressure and its complications of heart attack and stroke. Alcohol can cause irregularity of the heartbeat, known as atrial fibrillation, which in itself can increase the risk of clotting and stroke. Alcohol can directly damage the heart muscle itself causing a condition called cardiomyopathy, whereby the heart loses its ability to pump blood strongly; this can result in heart failure.

Cancers

Alcohol can increase the risk of many cancers, including cancer of the mouth and throat, and cancer of the oesophagus (food pipe), stomach, liver and pancreas gland. Excess alcohol may also have a role in increasing your risk of bowel or colon cancer as well as prostate cancer.

Alcohol and Liver Disease

The liver is the main organ responsible for filtering and removing alcohol from the body. The liver can metabolise and break down approximately 1 unit of alcohol per hour. However, if you drink alcohol faster than your liver can break it down then the amount of alcohol in your bloodstream rises.

Alcohol can affect the liver in three ways. Firstly, many people who drink excess alcohol develop what is known as a fatty liver. This is where you get a build-up of fat within the liver cells. Fatty liver is often reversible if you reduce your alcohol intake to within safe limits. However, sometimes people with fatty liver can go on to develop inflammation of the liver, known as alcoholic hepatitis.

Alcoholic hepatitis, secondly, is where the liver becomes swollen and inflamed. In mild cases this may not cause any symptoms and can simply be detected with a blood test, which may show an elevation of some of the liver enzymes. In more severe cases, though, you can feel unwell and develop nausea, yellow jaundice and sometimes pain over the liver area. If alcoholic hepatitis is severe, then the liver can shut down and go into liver failure, which can cause retention of fluid, life-threatening bleeding, confusion, coma and often death.

Finally, heavy drinking over a long period of time can lead to the development of alcoholic cirrhosis. Cirrhosis is a condition in which the normal soft, smooth tissue of the liver becomes replaced with hard, fibrous scar tissue. Some people who never drink alcohol can get cirrhosis, for example, as a result of viruses or other disorders of the immune system. However, it is felt that about one in ten heavy drinkers over a long period of time will get cirrhosis. Unfortunately, the scarring that occurs in the liver is irreversible. In severe cases, when the liver scarring is extensive, the only treatment option may be a liver transplant.

Muscles and Bones

Excess drinking can damage the muscles of the body, causing muscle wasting and reduced power. It can also cause a deficiency of calcium and thinning of the bones, which is known as osteoporosis.

Obesity

Alcohol can affect one's metabolism. It has the potential to be quite fattening. One gram of alcohol has 9 calories, which is the same amount of calories as 1 gram of fat. As well as that, alcohol has 'empty calories'. In other words, it has no nutritional value. This can lead to malnourishment through deficiency of valuable vitamins and minerals.

Alcohol stimulates the appetite, often causing men to consume more calories, for example, the trip to the chipper or a Chinese takeaway, which becomes more desirable after a few pints. Alcohol can trigger food cravings and compulsive eating patterns. This can clearly contribute to a bulging waistline and eventual obesity. It can also lead to a raised blood fat level (triglycerides), which can increase the risk of heart disease.

Digestive Tract

Alcohol can cause inflammation of the food pipe, causing heartburn or reflux of acid. It can damage the lining of the stomach, eroding it and sometimes aggravating stomach ulcers. This toxic effect on the gut wall can also lead to poor absorption of nutrients, which can contribute to malnutrition. Alcohol is one of the leading causes of pancreatitis, a painful condition caused by inflammation of the pancreas gland.

Immune System

Alcohol can affect the immune system and increase your risk of many immune-related disorders. A weakened immune system combined with malnutrition is one of the reasons why heavy drinking is associated with an increased risk of tuberculosis (TB). Alcohol can increase the risk of many infections, including pneumonia.

Blood

Alcohol affects the blood and can cause anaemia (low iron) and a low white cell count (the army that fights infection) as well as affecting the blood platelets and other blood-clotting factors, making bleeding more likely.

Sex Life

Excess alcohol can cause erectile dysfunction. As a depressive drug it will reduce libido. Alcohol can also lower the sperm count, contributing to male infertility.

Nervous System

Alcohol can damage the nerves and nervous system. It can damage nerves in the skin and legs, which can affect your ability to sense and touch objects. This is known as neuropathy. Alcohol can also damage the brain cells, leading to memory loss and confusion. Adolescents are thought to be particularly vulnerable to the effects of alcohol on the brain because their brains are still developing.

Chronic alcohol abuse can be associated with a form of dementia known as Korsakoff's syndrome, where the affected person has no short-term memory. There is a tendency to invent stories (known as confabulation) and in conversation a tendency to repeat the same stories over and over again. Long-term memory for distant events tends to remain good.

Alcohol can be associated with seizures, which are sometimes known as 'rum fits'. These seizures can occur a day or so after binge drinking as a response to withdrawal of the alcohol from the brain.

Mental Health

Alcohol can be associated with a long list of psychological health issues because it is a depressant. It can lower mood, leading to anxiety, panic and symptoms of depression. There is no doubt that many men who feel low turn to alcohol and drink more than they should. However this can make the depressive symptoms worse, which can cause a vicious cycle. As alcohol is a depressive drug it can lower your self esteem and diminish your get-up-and-go and zest for life. It can affect your sleep, particularly the quality of your sleep, so that the next day you feel tired.

Alcohol and Medication

Alcohol is a depressive drug and even one drink can impair judgment and reflexes. Alcohol has the potential to interact with a wide variety of other prescription medication. Some of these interactions can be potentially dangerous. For example, a well-known antibiotic called Flagyl (metronidazole) can cause you to become very unwell if you drink alcohol while on it. It is best to check with your doctor or pharmacist about any medication you have been prescribed, so you are aware of all the risks and can make an informed decision.

Social Costs of Alcohol

Alcohol is a major risk factor for accidents, including falls, fires and workplace accidents as well as road traffic accidents and death. This is because it affects reaction times, thought processing and coordination.

Drinking excessive amounts of alcohol can lead to unplanned sexual encounters, which can result in sexually transmitted infections and unplanned pregnancy, as well as regret and embarrassment. Alcohol can also encourage uninhibited behaviour patterns, resulting in overly emotional responses to certain situations. This can lead to aggression and potential violence.

Alcohol abuse is very much a family illness as all other family members can suffer as well. Alcohol can impair your performance as both a parent and a partner. Time spent drinking outside the home can compete with family time and the cost of alcohol can impact on needed resources for other family members. Alcohol abuse is also very much a part of the domestic violence story.

Alcohol is a major factor in work absenteeism, reduced productivity and poor job performance.

Health Benefits of Low-Dose Alcohol

For best health you should not drink more than 3 to 4 units on any one day. Binge drinking is dangerous and bad for your health. Social drinking is defined as using and enjoying alcohol in the context of a social occasion in the company of others, when alcohol is sipped and enjoyed slowly and you are aiming for no more than two to three drinks on that occasion. It is also suggested that a person should be free from or have a break from alcohol use for up to two to three days between social occasions.

There is a complex relationship between alcohol intake and heart disease. Compared to non-drinkers of alcohol, light to moderate drinkers, i.e. those who have one to two drinks per day, have a reduced risk of heart disease, heart attack and cardiac death. However, men who consume more than three drinks per day have an increased risk of heart disease and cardiac death.

How Does Alcohol Help the Heart?

It has been shown that alcohol increases the levels of HDL cholesterol, a protective type of cholesterol (see Chapter 6). One or two drinks per day can elevate your HDL cholesterol level by 5–10 per cent.

As well as that, some types of alcohol, particularly red wine, contains antioxidants such as flavinoids, which are thought to help prevent hardening of the arteries. Alcohol also has a beneficial effect on blood clotting by inhibiting the activity of platelets, which are part of the natural blood clotting process in the blood.

Alcohol and Risk of Death

Light to moderate drinking reduces the risk of angina, heart attack, ischemic stroke and sudden cardiac death. Overall, death rates seem to fall with light drinking but rise sharply as alcohol consumption increases. So, compared to non-drinkers, light drinkers live longer. However, as you drink more your risk of death increases rapidly, way above that of non-drinkers.

Other Benefits of Alcohol

Low-dose alcohol can help reduce the risk of developing diabetes and stroke. Low-dose alcohol may be pleasurable and relaxing, which may have important psychological and social benefits, and it may reduce your risk of developing erectile dysfunction.

What Is a Hangover?

A hangover is the physical after-effects of drinking excess alcohol. It is caused by toxins from alcohol and dehydration. The kidneys have to work much harder to clear alcohol from the body and as a result a lot of fluid is also lost, causing dehydration. Alcohol also reduces the supply of blood sugar from the liver, which results in lower blood sugar levels. The effects of this include feeling weak, fatigued and lightheaded. Cogeners can also contribute to a hangover. These are toxic chemicals produced as by-products during the fermentation of alcohol. Coloured drinks such as brandy, bourbon, red wine and champagne tend to have more congeners than clear drinks such as vodka or gin. Alcohol also can cause a deficiency of vitamins such as thiamine (Vitamin B_1).

How to Treat a Hangover

Symptoms of a hangover may include a pounding headache, nausea, dizziness and sensitivity to light and noise, all of which are self-inflicted. The best cure for a hangover is time, and the effects should go within 24 hours or so. However, the following will help:

- Drinking plenty of water will help combat the dehydrating effects of alcohol.
- Drinking fresh orange juice or eating lots of fresh fruit rich in Vitamin C is thought to help speed up the elimination of any residual alcohol in the system.
- One or two cups of coffee can also help.
- For hangover-induced headaches a mild pain killer such as paracetamol can be helpful. Celery juice or a tablespoon of honey can also help the headache.
- Milk thistle is thought to be a liver tonic, which can help the liver to clear alcohol from the body.

However prevention is clearly better than cure.

Self-Assessment Questionnaires Regarding Alcohol

CAGE Questionnaire

The CAGE questionnaire is a simple but quite accurate questionnaire that can detect your likelihood of alcohol dependency. It was developed by Dr John Ewing, founding director of the Bowles Center for

Alcohol Studies, University of North Carolina at Chapel Hill. The four questions are:

1. Have you ever tried to *cut* down on your drinking?
2. Have you ever been *annoyed* by criticism of your drinking?
3. Have you ever felt *guilty* about your drinking?
4. Have you ever had a morning *eye* opener?

Source: J.A. Ewing (1984), 'Detecting Alcoholism: The CAGE Questionnaire', *Journal of the American Medical Association*, 252: 1905–1907. Reproduced with permission.

Answering yes to one or more of these questions suggests that you may well be at risk of alcohol-related problems and that you may be better off avoiding alcohol.

AUDIT Questionnaire

The AUDIT questionnaire, also known as the Alcohol Use Disorders Identification Test, is another useful screening test to see if you are at risk of alcohol dependent problems. It was devised by and is copyright of the World Health Organization.

The AUDIT Questionnaire

1. How often do you have a drink containing alcohol?	
Never	0
Monthly or less	1
2 to 4 times per month	2
2 to 3 times per week	3
4 times or more per week	4
2. How many drinks do you have on a typical day when you are drinking?	
1 or 2	0
3 or 4	1
5 or 6	2
7 to 9	3
10 or more	4

(Continued)

3. How often do you have six or more drinks on one occasion?

Never	0
Less than monthly	1
Monthly	2
Weekly	3
Daily or almost daily	4

4. How often during the last year have you found that you were not able to stop drinking once you had started?

Never	0
Less than monthly	1
Monthly	2
Weekly	3
Daily or almost daily	4

5. How often during the last year have you failed to do what is normally expected from you because of drinking?

Never	0
Less than monthly	1
Monthly	2
Weekly	3
Daily or almost daily	4

6. How often during the last year have you needed a drink in the morning to get yourself going after a heavy drinking session?

Never	0
Less than monthly	1
Monthly	2
Weekly	3
Daily or almost daily	4

(Continued)

(Continued)

7. How often during the last year have you had a feeling of guilt or remorse after drinking?

Never	0
Less than monthly	1
Monthly	2
Weekly	3
Daily or almost daily	4

8. How often during the last year have you been unable to remember what happened the night before because you had been drinking?

Never	0
Less than monthly	1
Monthly	2
Weekly	3
Daily or almost daily	4

9. Have you or someone else been injured as a result of your drinking?

No	0
Yes, but not in the last year	2
Yes, during the last year	4

10. Has a relative, friend, doctor or other healthcare worker been concerned about your drinking or suggested you cut down?

No	0
Yes, but not in the last year	2
Yes, during the last year	4

Source: Babor, T.F., Higgins-Biddle, J.C., Saunders, J.B. and Monteiro, M.G. (2001), *AUDIT – The Alcohol Use Disorders Identification Test: Guidelines for Use in Primary Care*, Second edition, World Health Organization, Geneva. Reproduced with permission.

A score of 8 or higher on this questionnaire is considered positive and indicates that you are at risk of alcohol-related health difficulties.

Why Illegal Drugs Are Bad for Your Health

The use of illegal drugs has become widespread in the Western world in recent years and Ireland is no exception. The use and abuse of these substances is part of life in every corner of Ireland and not just in the bright lights of Dublin or Cork. Drugs can get into any household, irrespective of address, upbringing or bank balance. Educating yourself and your family about the real dangers of these substances is very important to dispel the myths that they are safe. Of course nothing could be further from the truth, as you will read below.

Cocaine

Cocaine is a white flaky powder made from the leaves of the coca plant, which grows in South America and South East Asia. 'Coke', 'white lady', 'snow' and 'gold dust' are just some of the street names for cocaine. In Ireland cocaine comes in two forms: cocaine powder and crack cocaine. Cocaine powder is usually used by snorting it through the nose. It is sometimes injected and can also be eaten. Crack cocaine is a more addictive form of cocaine and is usually smoked.

Cocaine used to be seen as an upper-class drug. However, since the Celtic Tiger years it has become much more widely available and for many people has become the illegal drug of choice. Regular and even daily use of cocaine is increasing. It is thought that about 7 per cent of Irish men have taken coke. In many ways the increase in cocaine usage has been a good analogy for the excesses of the Celtic Tiger and the 'I want it all and I'll have it all now' mentality. Attitudes to cocaine have accordingly changed with increased prosperity and the desire for instant gratification. Unfortunately, cocaine can have devastating effects on both physical and mental health and leave a trail of destruction in its wake

What Are the Effects of Cocaine?

Cocaine is a powerful stimulant drug and is highly addictive. The initial effects can include increased energy, confidence and alertness, and an increase in sex drive. The user may also feel less hungry, more aggressive, more excited and more prone to taking risks. Cocaine can also give you headaches, nausea and stomach or chest pains. Some users feel paranoid or suffer from hallucinations. As cocaine is used more often, tolerance develops, which means larger amounts of the drug are needed to achieve the same 'high' and the good feelings experienced tend to lessen. This can lead to serious adverse health effects. Cocaine is highly addictive and dependence (both physical and psychological) can develop rapidly, with strong cravings for cocaine.

Withdrawal effects can include sleep disturbance, exhaustion, irritability, restlessness and feelings of depression. Some people can experience severe seizures. 'Snow bugs' is an unpleasant crawling sensation that can be felt under the skin during cocaine withdrawal.

What Are the Medical Complications of Cocaine Abuse?

Cocaine is usually snorted into the nostrils. This causes the blood vessels in the nose to narrow, damaging the lining (septum) between both sides of the nose. Eventually a hole can appear in the septum. A tell-tale sign of regular cocaine use is a red, runny stuffed-up nose. Cocaine can also cause loss of smell, hoarseness and nosebleeds.

In the body cocaine causes the release of large amounts of the stress hormone noradrenaline, which causes the blood vessels in the body to narrow and your blood pressure to go up. As a result, some of the most frequent complications are effects on the heart. Cocaine can increase the heart rate, breathing and blood pressure. It can disrupt the electrical messages to the heart and bring on serious irregularities of the heart beat, called ventricular fibrillation. It can cause heart attacks and stroke.

The main blood vessel in the body, known as the aorta, can be damaged by cocaine use. This can lead to a tearing of the lining of the aorta, known as an aortic dissection. This tends to cause a crushing pain in the upper back or chest.

Cocaine can affect the lungs, causing chest pains, and sometimes the lungs may stop working. It can affect the brain, resulting in fever and headaches as well as strokes and seizures, and it can affect the stomach, causing abdominal pain and nausea. Chronic cocaine users can lose their appetites and become run-down, with accompanying weight loss. Eating cocaine can damage the blood supply to the bowel, resulting in gangrene.

Mental health effects are many and varied. Cocaine commonly causes anxiety, restlessness, panic attacks, depression and feelings of paranoia. This can lead to a paranoid psychosis where the person loses touch with reality and experiences auditory hallucinations (a sensation of hearing voices).

Regular users of cocaine can become impulsive and aggressive in their behaviour and lose their sense of perspective. This can lead to more violence and risk-taking, for example when driving.

Mixing Cocaine and Alcohol

There is a potentially dangerous interaction between cocaine and alcohol. Taken in combination, the two drugs are converted by the body to cocaethylene. Alcohol makes cocaine last longer because of the way the drugs interact in the liver. Mixing cocaine and alcohol significantly increases the risk of heart attack.

Cannabis

What Is Cannabis?

The cannabis plant contains many different chemicals and can come in many different strengths, with variable effects. The plant is used as either the resin (a brownish/black lump) or as herbal cannabis, which is made from the dried leaves and flowering tops. Other names for cannabis include 'marijuana', 'weed', 'puff', 'hash' and 'wacky backy'. Cannabis is usually taken by mixing it with tobacco. It is then inhaled deeply into the lungs for a number of seconds. Cannabis can also be smoked in a pipe and can be brewed as tea or even cooked as 'hash cakes'.

How Does It Work?

Cannabis affects special areas of the brain called cannabinoid receptors, which are mainly found in areas of the brain that influence pleasure, thoughts, and sensory and time perception.

Cannabis gets into the bloodstream quickly after being taken and tends to build up in fatty tissues throughout the body. It is stored there and it can take several weeks for the body to eliminate it. This is why cannabis can sometimes be detected in urine up to 56 days after it has last been used.

What Are Its Effects?

Short-term use of cannabis can affect people in different ways. These can include a temporary 'high', a sense of relaxation or contentment (of being 'stoned'), becoming more talkative and sometimes having a sense of time slowing down. Changes in awareness can make colours seem more intense and music sound better. Cravings for food (having the 'munchies') and hallucinations (when you see or hear something that isn't there) may occur. Short-term memory, concentration and learning can be affected. Cannabis can also cause feelings of nausea, fatigue and loss of energy and can affect your coordination. The feelings are usually only temporary, although the drug can stay in the system for some weeks.

Long-term cannabis use can have a depressant effect, reducing motivation and leading to apathy. Short-term memory, concentration and learning can be affected. This can lead to poor performance at work or school.

Health Risks of Cannabis

Smoking cannabis damages your throat and lungs just like cigarettes do. It can cause hoarseness, a chronic cough and bronchitis as well as lung damage, including lung cancer. Indeed, smoking cannabis is thought to be even worse for your lungs than cigarettes. Cannabis can affect male fertility by leading to a decreased sperm count and reduced sperm mobility.

Mental health problems can include confusion, anxiety, panic, depression, paranoia and schizophrenia. Regular use of the drug increases the risk of developing a psychotic episode or long-term schizophrenia.

Speed

Speed (amphetamine) is a man-made stimulant that is usually swallowed in pill form. It can also be a powder that is dissolved in liquid for injection or drinking. Amphetamine is a stimulant, which quickens the heartbeat and can increase energy levels, making the user feel more confident. It can also cause anxiety, panic and paranoia, as well as impaired memory and concentration. The 'come down' period, when the effects wear off, can last for days, with users feeling very tired and depressed and having symptoms of anxiety and panic.

Sleep disturbance is very common and can keep users awake for days afterwards.

Speed can increase your blood pressure, which can cause a stroke. Regular users can become very run-down with a weakened immune system, which makes them more prone to all types of infections. Mental health can be severely affected by regular use, leading to severe depression and paranoia, with an increased risk of psychosis.

Ecstasy

Ecstasy is made up of a mixture of substances, including a synthetic drug called MDMA, and is classed as a hallucinogenic amphetamine. It comes in tablet form and is swallowed. Other names for ecstasy include 'E', 'doves', 'XTC' and 'disco biscuits'. Taking ecstasy can cause relaxation, disinhibition and feelings of warmth. It is sometimes known as the 'love drug'. Initial effects can last for several hours and include feeling more alert; colours, sound and emotions can also seem more intense. Feelings of confusion, anxiety and paranoia may occur. The 'come down' phase can cause profound fatigue, inability to sleep and feelings of depression.

Health risks include blurred vision, liver and kidney problems and a danger of overheating and getting dehydrated if you are out dancing in a club. This is known as 'heat stroke' due to a combination of a raised body temperature from the ecstasy and dehydration from dancing and the rise in temperature. It can lead to convulsions, coma or even heart attack and stroke. Heart palpitations can occur with an increase in blood pressure and skin temperature. Mental health problems include long-term damage to serotonin receptors in the brain with an increased risk of depression.

Heroin

Heroin is made from the pain-killing drug morphine and comes from the opium plant. It is a highly addictive drug with tolerance developing rapidly so that users need to take more and more heroin to get the same 'high'. Heroin can be smoked, sniffed or injected. When you take heroin there is an intense rush of excitement followed by a dream-like state of relaxation. These effects can last several hours and are much more intense if the heroin is injected. First time use, especially if injected, often causes nausea, vomiting and severe headaches. Sharing needles when injecting heroin increases the risk of blood-acquired infections such as blood poisoning or HIV, and Hepatitis B and C. Withdrawal symptoms can occur within 24 hours of the last 'fix' and include a multitude of symptoms known collectively as 'cold turkey'. These can include sweats, chills, anxiety, irritability, cramps and muscle spasms.

The use of heroin can lead to significant health problems. These include a weakened immune system from poor nutrition, collapsed veins, skin abscesses, an increased risk of pneumonia and other chest problems, and chronic constipation. Using heroin can affect your fertility and cause erectile dysfunction. The drug can consume a user's life, leading to the breakdown of relationships, career and home life. Many addicts get involved in crime to feed their habit. Heroin can lead to mental health problems, including depression and suicide.

LSD (Acid)

LSD is a hallucinogenic drug that comes either in pill form or embedded in a small piece of paper. It changes the way in which the mind perceives colour, sound, events and time, and this experience is called a 'trip'. This can be a pleasant experience (good trip) or it can be very frightening, with feelings of panic and paranoia (bad trip). It can lead to long-term mental health problems. Flashbacks can occur in some people up to months after taking acid, whereby the experiences of the 'trip' return temporarily.

Tranquilisers (Sedatives)

Sedatives are drugs that are used medically to help induce sleep or as a short-term option to treat severe stress or anxiety. However, they can also be misused and abused due to their widespread 'recreational' or non-medical use. People who have difficulty dealing with stress, anxiety or sleeplessness may overuse or become dependent on sedatives. Sedatives are also widely abused by other drug takers. For example, heroin users may take them either as a substitute or to supplement their heroin use. Stimulant users may take sedatives to calm feelings of edginess. Others take sedatives to relax and forget their worries. These drugs include diazepam (Valium), nitrazepam (Mogadon) and temazepam (Normison).

Accidental overdose with sedatives can occur when someone who is drowsy or confused repeats the dose. Mixing sedatives with alcohol is dangerous as the two drugs can combine to slow brain function and breathing, leading to loss of consciousness and even death. Sometimes sedative use can bring on symptoms of depression, aggressive behaviour, phobias and other mental health problems. Sedatives can sometimes cause long-term or short-term memory problems.

Magic Mushrooms

Magic mushrooms are mushrooms that grow wild, usually in October and November. They are hallucinogenic and can be eaten raw, cooked or made into a tea. Their effects are similar to a mild LSD trip. They can cause symptoms of relaxation and excitement as well as hallucinations and paranoia. Magic mushrooms increase blood pressure and heart rate and after eating them you can get dizzy and nauseous. Flashbacks can occur and taking them can lead to mental health problems.

Solvents

Solvent abuse is not only glue sniffing but the sniffing of any substance that contains butane or propane gas – aerosols, gas refills and paint thinners are a few examples. The result is a 'high' similar to that produced by alcohol. Like alcohol you get a hangover afterwards. The inhalation has potentially serious side-effects, including sudden death due to effects on the heart, lungs or brain. Death can occur on the very first occasion of use. Accidents can occur when using solvents, including suffocation and inhalation of vomit.

Getting Help

If you think alcohol or drugs may be having a negative effect on your life, you are not alone. Addiction is all too common among Irish men. The first step to recovery is admitting to yourself that you may have a problem and accepting the need to make changes. Talk to your family doctor, who can support you and give you help and advice. Your doctor may refer you for counselling. AA (Alcoholics Anonymous) and NA (Narcotics Anonymous) can provide group support through regular meetings. Specialised addiction centres like Aiseiri can provide great residential recovery programmes with an aftercare follow-up plan. Unfortunately, many Irish men remain in denial.

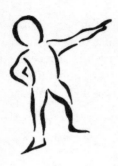

Key Points

- Alcohol is a potentially serious health hazard for many Irish men.
- Abuse of alcohol often results in mental health issues, including anxiety and depression. Physically, almost every part of your body can be affected by alcohol, including your sexual health.
- Irish men often drink more than is good for their health.
- Alcohol is measured in units and there is a tendency to underestimate the number of units consumed.
- Keeping a diary of your drinking habits for a week or two (including weekends or nights out) can help give you an accurate picture of your level of consumption.
- Self-assessment questionnaires can help you decide if you are drinking too much for your health. If you don't ask an honest question you won't get an honest answer.
- Making a decision to reduce your alcohol intake can be very positive for your health, as well as your wallet and waistline.
- The taking of illegal drugs such as cannabis and cocaine is now widespread among Irish men. These substances can have serious ill effects on your physical and mental health.
- Recreational illegal drugs, by their nature, mess with your mind – that's partly the idea. They can also have serious effects on your long-term physical and mental health. Be warned!
- There is a lot of help out there if you feel alcohol or drugs are having negative effects on your health. Talk to your family doctor, who will help and advise you.

14

Stress and Distress

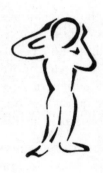

What Is Stress?

Stress is a very normal human reaction to a perceived threat from any source. A certain amount of stress in our lives is good for all of us. Stress can mean different things to different people. It can have a positive and a negative effect. Stress can be positive when it motivates us to get things done that are important to us. However, it can be negative when we constantly feel pressurised or traumatised by too many demands.

Without some stress we could not get out of bed in the morning, never mind do a day's work. However, when we are under too much stress or when the stress we are under exceeds our ability to cope, stress can turn into 'distress'. By distress I mean that the level of stress we are under is having a negative effect on us. This can be bad for both our short- and long-term health, with potential adverse health consequences.

What Happens to Our Bodies When We Are Under Stress?

Stress wakens up or arouses our system, so that we experience the 'fight or flight' response. At a primitive level this meant that when a caveman was walking in the woods and came across a big brown bear his body could make very quick adjustments so that he could take drastic action and save himself from the bear.

The heart starts to beat faster and pump more blood, raising the blood pressure. The pupils (the dark parts) of the eyes widen to allow in more light, the breathing gets faster and the tubes going into the lungs widen to let in more oxygen, the mind becomes more alert, blood is diverted towards the muscles, which become tense and ready for action, while blood is diverted away from the gut and the skin, which becomes cold and clammy. As well as that, hormones called adrenaline and cortisol are pumped into the blood, which causes the blood sugar to rise providing an immediate source of energy. Changes also occur in the blood, enabling it to clot more easily – a basic protective mechanism to enable quick repair of any wounds. All of these changes happen very quickly, allowing our caveman to fight or take flight. In the case of our brown bear, his best option is to leg it as fast as he can.

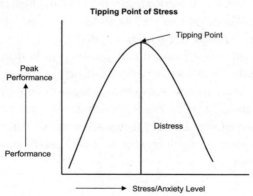

256

So, as you can see, stress is an essential and very useful mechanism by which the body and mind can adapt to rapidly changing circumstances. Stress can be good for our health and welfare and is a necessary tool for survival.

You can see from the diagram (above) that a certain amount of stress increases performance; however, once the amount of stress we are under goes beyond a certain point, known as the 'tipping point', then performance actually starts to reduce with increasing amounts of stress. In this situation we are in a state of distress, which can be very harmful to our health. The amount of stress we can individually cope with varies from person to person. This may tend to depend at least partly on personality, but also on our own coping mechanisms for dealing with stress.

Studies also show that men and women handle stress differently. This may in part be due to biological reasons. Also, men often don't have the strong social support networks that women have to turn to during times of stress. These social supports may help explain why women, in general, seem to be better able to cope with stress than men.

Modern life can be stressful and Irish men seem to have become increasingly susceptible to stress and other mental health problems. Large numbers of Irish men suffer from stress, but often in silence. Irish men are slow to seek help with mental health issues, including stress. This may be for many reasons, including ignorance, fear, embarrassment or the perception that admitting to being stressed in some way implies inadequacy or weakness. It goes back to the attitude that 'real' men don't go to the doctor and that big boys don't cry. Unfortunately this type of attitude does nothing to help Irish men or their loved ones.

Is Stress Harmful?

The precise mechanisms that govern the interactions between stress and ill-health remain poorly understood. However, it is felt that chronic stress can affect the quality of the immune system, causing the body's own natural defences against illness to be lowered. One possible explanation for this is that prolonged job stress may affect the nervous system. Another possible reason for this is the fact that chronic stress may affect the body's hormonal balance and result in a weakened immune system.

Chronic stress is a risk factor for heart disease. Research has found a link between chronic stress and the development of heart disease, type 2 diabetes and metabolic syndrome. Metabolic syndrome is the presence of three or more of the following five factors: high blood pressure, central obesity (excessive abdominal fat), raised blood fat (triglycerides), low HDL cholesterol (see Chapter 6) and raised blood sugar.

Chronic stress is also associated with many other medical conditions, including:

- Irritable bowel syndrome
- Migraine
- Psoriasis
- Tension headaches
- High blood pressure
- Some cancers
- Depression
- Hair loss
- Diabetes
- Ulcers
- Burnout
- Heart disease and stroke

Stress and Heart Disease

Chronic stress – or rather distress – is thought to be a risk factor for heart disease in later life. Anger and hostility can be powerful emotions with the potential to trigger a heart attack.

The link between stress and heart disease is complex and not fully understood. If you feel stressed, your body will produce more stress hormones. Although they are useful in small quantities, too much of these hormones, continuously and over time, can damage your arteries and may lead to high blood pressure. Also, when life becomes pressurised, people are more likely to smoke more cigarettes, drink more caffeine, drink too much alcohol and be less physically active. All of these things can contribute to heart problems.

Symptoms and Signs of Stress in Irish Men

Your relationships and your performance at work, at home and in the bedroom can all be affected by excess stress. Telltale signs of stress building up include some or all of the following symptoms:

- Feeling tense – this may include a knot in the stomach or neck and shoulder tension
- Feeling sweaty or having a dry mouth
- Being unable to make decisions
- Reduced work performance
- Sleep disturbance
- Loss of enjoyment of food
- Loss of interest in hobbies
- Being irritable or impatient, short-tempered or snappy
- Constipation and/or diarrhoea
- Increased need to urinate
- Feeling tired all the time, fatigue
- Heartburn

- Headaches
- Being more withdrawn, less sociable
- Having a constant need to stay busy
- Increased alcohol intake
- Erectile dysfunction

The Type A Personality

'One man's meat is another mans' poison', as the saying goes. What's stressful to one man may be all in a day's work for another. The difference appears to lie in our perceptions of various events. It is felt that personality can play a major role in how we perceive and cope with stress.

Many factors influence and shape our character. These include a large inbuilt or genetic component. We have our own unique temperament when we are born. This is further influenced by our life's experiences, which affects our individual way of thinking, feeling and behaving. This is your personality.

Men with 'Type A' personalities, for example, tend to be in a hurry, ambitious, time-conscious and driven. These traits, if not properly managed, can create stress-related illnesses.

On the other hand, men with 'Type B' personalities are much more relaxed, and less time-conscious and driven. Type B personalities are better able to put things into perspective, and think through how they are going to deal with situations. Consequently, they tend to be less prone to the adverse effects of stress.

Type A Personality Traits

The term 'Type A personality' has become a household phrase over the past fifty years. Type A behaviour includes time urgency, impatience, rudeness and 'having a short fuse'. Additionally, Type A behaviour often includes competitiveness and a strong orientation towards high achievement.

Physical characteristics that can result from years of chronic stress and Type A behaviour include teeth grinding, tight lips and a clenched jaw.

Negative Effects of Type A Behaviour

Over the years, the extra stress that most Type A people experience takes a toll on their health and lifestyle. Type A men usually find themselves in stressful, demanding occupations (and sometimes the jobs create the Type A behaviour), which can lead to health problems. The following are some of the negative effects that are common among those exhibiting Type A behaviour:

- Hypertension – high-blood pressure is more common among Type A personalities.
- Heart disease – the risk of heart disease is increased in men with Type A behaviour.
- Social isolation – these men often spend too much time on work and focus too little on relationships. The emphasis is mainly on the urgent things like work, at the expense of family, hobbies and personal development. This attitude puts them at risk of social isolation, the increased stress that comes with it and eventual potential burnout.

Burnout

Burnout is a term used to describe someone who is completely mentally and physically exhausted. Chronic stress can cause burnout, so that a person becomes emotionally exhausted and feels a strong lack of personal accomplishment. There are many early warning signs of burnout:

- Chronic fatigue – exhaustion, tiredness, a sense of being physically rundown
- A sense of being besieged
- Anger at those making demands
- Self-criticism for putting up with the demands
- Cynicism, negativity and irritability
- Losing your temper easily over seemingly trivial things
- Feelings of helplessness
- Increased degree of risk-taking
- Physical symptoms, which may include frequent headaches, gastrointestinal disturbances, weight changes, sleep disturbance and symptoms of depression

Stress Busters

The good news is that there are several things you can do to stay healthy and reverse many of the negative effects of stress in a surprisingly short amount of time, with a few relatively minor lifestyle changes. Men who cope best with stress seem to have these things in common:

- A sense of being in control of their lives
- A network of friends or family to provide social support
- Personality traits like flexibility and hopefulness

There is no doubt a healthy lifestyle can protect against the adverse effects of stress. A good, regular exercise programme, combined with a healthy diet and adequate relaxation time, can be a great counterbalance to a stressful job. Getting enough sleep and maintaining a positive outlook are also important for overall health.

Stress management is a life skill which we men can learn. While there is no such thing as a one-size-fits-all solution, the following list of stress busters can help combat the adverse effects of stress.

Get in Touch with Your Emotions

- Talk about your feelings. This can be difficult for us men as it's often something we find difficult and may have little experience of.
- Don't bottle up your emotions. Learn to express and talk through your feelings. Writing your feelings down can be an excellent way of letting off steam, even if the letter gets shredded at the end.
- Build and develop your relationships.

Reduce Daily Stressors by Taking Control – Change What You Can

Even men with the most adaptable personalities can experience the effects of long-term stress if they lack a sense of control over aspects of their daily lives. You can reduce stress in your life by making lifestyle changes like becoming more organised and better at managing time, rather than allowing time to manage you.

Time Management

- Keep a weekly planner so that you can prioritise things that are important to you such as family and down time. In other words, make time for the non-urgent.
- Learn to prioritise and learn to delegate
- Learn to say 'NO'

Lifestyle Choices

- Eat a healthy diet

- Drink plenty of water.
- Respect alcohol – many men drink excess alcohol when under stress.
- Avoid stimulants in your diet, particularly excess caffeine. Cut out or cut down on your coffee intake. Switch some cups to decaf. Similarly with tea, which has a surprisingly high caffeine content. Three to four mugs of tea a day is plenty of caffeine for all of us. Avoid caffeine late in the evening as this can interfere with your sleep pattern. Consider trying some green tea; it is delicious, caffeine-free and full of antioxidants: three good reasons to enjoy it.
- Work off stress – physical activity helps to produce the body's own 'happy' hormones, or antidepressants, called endorphins. These give us that feel-good factor we experience after exercise. Be more active everyday. Walk briskly, cycle, jog, swim or enjoy any favourite activity for at least 30 minutes.

Enjoy Yourself

- Have a laugh – serious thinking and behaviour can cause stress, whereas laughter can uncork the pressure and release built-up tension. Laughing also helps us get a better view of the problem and tends to make us feel more light-hearted.
- Have a treat – whenever you are faced with a difficult challenge, plan to give yourself a treat afterwards. Having something to look forward to will help you cope much better.

Consider Relaxation Techniques

These can help your health by activating your body's relaxation response (the mechanism in your body that counteracts the 'fight or flight' response to stress, helping hormone levels and other systems to return to normal):

- Learn to properly relax. Consider yoga, tai chi, reflexology or therapeutic massage.
- Massage – massage can ease aches and pains, and help your body relax and unwind.
- Breathing exercises can be excellent for emotional calming. Practise this every day:
  - sit in a comfortable position on a chair with a good back support
  - make sure both feet are firmly on the ground
  - close your eyes
  - put your hands on your thighs with the palms facing upwards
  - slowly count from one to four as you breathe in through your nose
  - pause for two counts
  - then open your mouth and mentally count from one to six as you breathe out through your mouth
  - continue this slow rhythmic breathing for several minutes
  - slowly open your eyes and sit quietly

How Much Stress Am I Under?

To measure stress according to the Holmes and Rahe Stress Scale, the number of 'life change units' that apply to events in the past year of an individual's life are added and the final score will give a rough estimate of how stress affects health.

Holmes and Rahe Stress Scale

Life Event	Life Change Units
Death of a spouse	100
Divorce	73
Marital separation	65
Imprisonment	63
Death of a close family member	63
Personal injury or illness	53
Marriage	50
Dismissal from work	47
Marital reconciliation	45
Retirement	45
Change in health of a family member	44
Pregnancy	40
Sexual difficulties	39
Gain a new family member	39
Business readjustment	39
Change in financial state	38
Change in frequency of arguments	35
Major mortgage	32
Foreclosure of mortgage or loan	30
Change in responsibilities at work	29
Child leaving home	29
Trouble with in-laws	29
Outstanding personal achievement	28
Spouse starts or stops work	26
Begin or end school	26
Change in living conditions	25
Revision of personal habits	24
Trouble with boss	23

(Continued)

(Continued)

Life Event	Life Change Units
Change in working hours or conditions	20
Change in residence	20
Change in schools	20
Change in recreation	19
Change in church activities	19
Change in social activities	18
Minor mortgage or loan	17
Change in sleeping habits	16
Change in number of family reunions	15
Change in eating habits	15
Vacation	13
Christmas	12
Minor violation of the law	11

Reprinted from the *Journal of Psychosomatic Research*, Vol. 11, No. 2, Holmes, T.H., Rahe, R.H., 'The Social Readjustment Rating Scale', pp. 213–218, © 1967, with permission from Elsevier.

Score of 300+: At risk of stress-induced illness
Score of 150–299+: Risk of stress-induced illness is moderate (reduced by 30 per cent from the above risk)
Score of less than 150: Only have a slight risk of stress-induced illness

Anxiety

Anxiety is an unpleasant condition characterised by a tendency to worry excessively. It can occur in up to 8 per cent of Irish men. This excessive worry is accompanied by physical symptoms, such as sweaty hands, irritability, restlessness, bowel symptoms such as wind, light-headedness, muscle tension and aches. Anxiety disorder can bring on physical illness and it has been associated with an increased risk of heart disease in particular. It can lead to alcohol abuse or other substance abuse. The key to treating and managing anxiety is to first recognise it exists. Keep a detailed symptom diary for a week or so.

Anxiety can be a prominent symptom of clinical depression, so if you are a man and feel anxious you should have a good chat with your family doctor, who will be able to help you decide if it is lifestyle factors, adverse effects of alcohol, anxiety disorder, clinical depression or a combination of all of the above that are contributing to your symptoms.

Treatment

Keeping a detailed lifestyle diary for a week or two, including everything you eat and drink, your exercise levels and your perceived levels of stress, can give you a very useful insight into the role your lifestyle is playing in your symptoms.

Exercise can be an excellent way to combat the effects of stress and get rid of tension. It can often be worth quitting alcohol for a month or so to see what effect that has on your physical and mental well-being. At the very least, keep your alcohol intake within recommended limits (no more than 21 units per week, of which no more than 4 units per day). Minimise your intake of stimulants such as caffeine.

Relaxation exercises, including deep breathing and meditation, can be very helpful for stress also. Counselling can sometimes be very effective for anxiety. Your doctor may prescribe some medication for you, particularly if he feels you are lacking in serotonin. The following are some tricks and techniques to help you de-stress.

- Follow the breathing exercise outlined above.
- Practice smiling.
- Try not to clench your teeth.

- Talk slowly.
- Try not to interrupt.
- Eat slowly and always eat at the table.
- Monitor your use of language.
- Don't permit outbursts of anger. If you feel upset about something, pause, reflect and take deep breaths. Express yourself calmly.

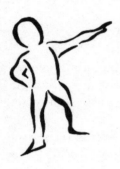

Key Points

- Some stress is necessary for us to function and is part and parcel of life for Irish men.
- However, excess stress – or distress – can have adverse consequences for both our physical and mental health.
- Chronic stress is associated with many physical health conditions, including heart disease.
- Mental health issues such as depression and burnout may result from chronic stress.
- Being able to de-stress is important for our well-being.
- Proactive stress management techniques can be an invaluable life skill for Irish men.

15

Depression

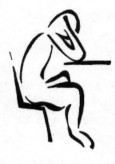 Depression is common among Irish men and is often undiagnosed. Men tend to bottle up feelings, suppress and internalise emotions, and suffer stoically in silence. The natural resistance of the Irish male to seek help is compounded further by his general reluctance to discuss mental health issues. Some men still perceive depression to be a stigma, implying weakness or inadequacy. Nothing, however, could be further from the truth.

Unlike women, men are usually unable to articulate their feelings through their support networks or friends. Yet it is only through education and by increasing awareness of the symptoms, causes of and treatments for depression that we can help to bridge the gap that currently exists in Irish society for Irish men. Undiagnosed and untreated depression in severe forms can increase the risk of suicide, which is tragically all too common amongst Irish men, particularly young men.

Check out the self-assessment test for depression at the end of this chapter and see how you fare out. If you think you may be suffering from symptoms of depression, don't suffer in silence. Your family doctor is there to help and support you.

Some Facts

- One in every four Irish men will develop depression at some time in their lives.
- Suicide is at least four times more common in men than women.
- The majority of suicides can be traced back to depression.
- Suicide is the biggest killer of young men aged 15–24.

Types of Depression

Depression is a medical condition caused by a chemical imbalance in the brain, usually a deficiency of serotonin (the happy hormone). This can occur as a reaction to a major, often traumatic, life event or to chronic stress. This type of depression is known as reactive depression.

I have often heard it said, 'sure he has nothing to be depressed about.' But sometimes depression can occur without there being any underlying reason and this is known as endogenous depression. This can affect anyone, irrespective of upbringing, address or bank balance.

Bipolar disorder, which used to be called 'manic depression', is a much less common condition. This is where episodes of elation or mania alternate with bouts of depression.

What Are the Symptoms of Depression?

Temporary feelings of sadness or depression are part of the normal ups and downs of everyday life. Clinical depression is more than that. Some or all of the following symptoms may be present:

- A low mood every day or most days for at least two weeks
- Loss of enjoyment or interest in usual activities, particularly things you would normally enjoy, like hobbies
- Lack of motivation, or 'get up and go'. Sometimes even simple tasks can seem difficult.
- Difficulty concentrating, for example, when reading and at work
- Sleep difficulties: difficulty getting to sleep, difficulty staying asleep or early morning wakening. Classically, this early morning wakening occurs when you wake up early but are unable to get back to sleep, and yet you still feel tired. Sometimes people with depression can oversleep.
- Feelings of sadness, sometimes with tearfulness
- Feelings of guilt
- Feelings of hopelessness or worthlessness
- Lack of energy
- Loss of interest in sex
- Erectile dysfunction
- Lack of emotion
- Change in appetite: this is usually a loss of interest in and taste for food with associated weight loss. However, sometimes comfort or binge eating can occur with subsequent weight gain.
- Feelings of irritability, agitation or restlessness
- Mood variation during the day, with symptoms often worse early in the day
- Physical symptoms including headaches, constipation, palpitations, fatigue or feeling tired all the time
- Thoughts of death, which may include passive death wishes, where someone feels they would be better off dead
- A feeling of 'blackness'
- Occasional suicidal thoughts

As a general rule, the more of the above symptoms you have the more severe the depression. More severe forms of depression, particularly when associated with feelings of hopelessness about the future or worthlessness, can be associated with an increased risk of suicide.

Specific Medical Criteria for the Diagnosis of Major Depression

Symptoms of depression must be present nearly every day for at least two weeks and not explained by medical conditions, strokes or recent bereavement.

At least one of these two symptoms should be present:

- Depressed mood

OR

- Severely diminished interest in or pleasure from activities that are usually pleasurable

In addition, at least four of the following seven symptoms should be present:

- Substantial change in appetite or weight loss or, less commonly, weight gain
- Inability to sleep or, less commonly, excessive sleep
- Fatigue or loss of energy
- Diminished physical activity or, less commonly, agitation
- Impaired ability to think, concentrate or make decisions
- Diminished self-esteem, with feelings of worthlessness or inappropriate guilt
- Recurrent thoughts of death or suicide

What Causes Depression?

Depression is thought to occur when there is a chemical imbalance in the brain. Men suffering from depression are thought to have lower levels of some of the chemical messengers in the brain, called neurotransmitters. The three neurotransmitters believed to be involved in depression are serotonin, dopamine and noradrenaline. It is thought that, when levels of serotonin or the other brain chemicals drop, then symptoms of depression kick in. This fall in neurotransmitter levels can occur without there being any obvious reason. Just like the man who eats a healthy diet can still have high cholesterol, the man without any obvious underlying cause can develop symptoms of depression. However, stressful life events such as losing your job, relationship difficulties or illness can also trigger depression.

Some Medical Causes of Depression

- Chronic pain from any cause
- Chronic illness, including lung problems, diabetes, cancer, multiple sclerosis, heart disease, metabolic disorders and thyroid problems
- Substance abuse – alcohol, cocaine or other drugs
- Withdrawal from stimulants, including nicotine and caffeine
- Medications including beta blockers, steroids, pain killers, sleeping tablets and antihistamines
- Neurological conditions like Alzheimer's disease and other forms of dementia, stroke, brain tumours, Parkinson's disease, multiple sclerosis and seizure disorders such as epilepsy
- Infections such as flu, glandular fever, Lyme disease (from tick bites) and HIV

Treatment of Depression

It is well recognised that a healthy lifestyle has a positive effect on mood and mental health generally. Regular exercise is thought to have a mood-elevating effect by stimulating the release of the happy hormone serotonin. A healthy diet and lifestyle is conducive to good mental health and will help the recovery process. Eating plenty of fresh fruit and vegetables, wholegrains and oily fish, and drinking plenty of water is also good for your health in general. Depression recovery begins with building supportive relationships and challenging any negative thoughts. Also, minding your physical health will slowly but surely lift your mental health. Treatment can involve counselling/talking therapy or medication, or a combination of both.

Talking Therapy or Counselling

This can be helpful if there is an underlying stressful issue causing your depression, for example, a relationship difficulty. Individual counselling therapy, marital and family counselling, or group therapy can all be helpful ways of treating depressive symptoms. This process can allow you the opportunity to learn healthier ways of dealing with negative feelings and solving problems. It is important that you go to a suitably trained and qualified counsellor. The Irish Association of Counselling Therapists (IACT) is a useful place to find someone suitable in your area, or ask your GP for advice.

Cognitive Behavioural Therapy

This is based on the idea that, by changing the way you think, feel and behave, you can eliminate mental health problems such as depression. The aim is to make your thought patterns more realistic and helpful. This type of treatment is generally done in weekly sessions over several months. Psychotherapy can help you get to the root of your problems and change your negative thinking patterns, and allows you to learn new ways of coping.

Antidepressant Medication

Medication can be helpful in treating depression by correcting any underlying serotonin imbalance in the brain. It is not addictive and can take up to four to six weeks to kick in. A normal course of therapy is for about six months. While people may feel better after a few weeks and may be inclined to stop the treatment, this significantly increases the chance of a relapse. This is no different to being given a seven-day course of an antibiotic for a chest infection; you may feel better after two or three days, but if you do not finish the course there is a good chance your infection may come back.

Unfortunately, some men remain resistant to the idea of taking antidepressant medication, even though it can work well and is relatively safe. Very few men would argue about the need for a plaster of Paris if they fell and broke their leg. Why should treating depression be any different?

<u>Types of Antidepressants</u>

There are several different types of antidepressant medication available and these are discussed briefly below.

SSRIs (Selective Serotonin Reuptake Inhibitors)

The SSRIs are the most commonly prescribed class of antidepressant. They increase the level of serotonin available in the brain. The SSRIs include drugs such as fluoxetine (Prozac), escitalopram (Lexapro) and sertraline (Lustral). The SSRIs are usually preferred over older classes of antidepressants, such as tricyclic antidepressants and

MAOIs, because their adverse effects are less severe. Common side effects of SSRIs include nausea, sleep disturbance and anxiety. Other recognised side effects include dizziness, headaches, dry mouth, sweating, tremors, weight gain and constipation or diarrhoea. Sexual side effects are also common with SSRIs, such as a decreased sex drive (reduced libido), trouble reaching orgasm (known as anorgasmia) and erectile problems. These sexual side effects usually reverse on stopping the drug.

Newer Atypical Antidepressants

These medications target other brain chemicals such as noradrenaline and dopamine as well as serotonin. Side effects can include nausea, drowsiness or tiredness, weight gain, dry mouth, anxiety and blurred vision. Examples of these drugs include venlafaxine (Efexor) and mirtazapine (Zispin).

Tricyclic Antidepressants

Tricyclics are among the oldest antidepressants. They tend to cause more side effects than the others. Drowsiness is a common side effect. Other common side effects include dry mouth, blurred vision, dizziness, tremors, sexual problems and weight gain. Examples include amitriptyline (Tryptizol) and clomipramine (Anafranil).

MAOIs (Monoamine Oxidase Inhibitors)

MAOIs have severe interactions with certain foods, drinks and medications containing tyramine, such as chocolate, cheese and alcohol. This can result in dangerously high blood pressure, which can lead to a stroke or heart attack. For this reason these drugs are not commonly used. An example of an MAOI is tranylcypromine (Parnate).

Antidepressant Withdrawal

While antidepressant medication is not addictive, it is not a good idea to stop it suddenly. If you do, you may experience a number of unpleasant withdrawal symptoms known as antidepressant discontinuation syndrome. These symptoms may include flu-like symptoms, nausea, anxiety, restlessness, agitation and sleep disturbance, including nightmares. Therefore, as with all medication, it is important to discuss any potential changes with your doctor.

How Effective Are Antidepressants?

Treatment with antidepressant medication can help about 70 per cent of people with depression. Some people can't tolerate the side effects. There are sometimes other effective treatment approaches that can be taken in addition to or instead of medications. It's up to you to evaluate your options and decide what's best for you. A good chat with your family doctor is a great place to start. Being aware of the facts can help you make an informed and personal decision about how best to treat your depression.

St John's Wort

St John's wort has been shown to be effective in treating mild depression. Otherwise known as *Hypericum perforatum*, the plant's common name comes from the fact that its flowers typically bloom around the birthday of St John the Baptist on 24 June each year. St John's wort is used widely throughout Europe and America to treat symptoms of anxiety, stress and mild depression. It is sometimes referred to as 'nature's Prozac'. Many people like the fact that it is a natural product and may be more amenable to trying this rather than conventional medication. In many countries, St John's wort is available in health shops as a supplement. However, here in Ireland it is only available on prescription. There is some evidence that it can be effective in treating mild depression, helping to raise serotonin levels. The active ingredient is hypericin and there can be a wide range of potency and purity in the preparations available.

It appears to be safe, with few side effects. Some people describe stomach upset, tiredness, dry mouth or dizziness when using it. However, it does increase the tendency to sunburn, if you are fortunate enough to experience some good weather. St John's wort can interfere with other medications, including warfarin, drug treatments for epilepsy, depression and heart disease, antibiotics and over-the-counter cough bottles such as pseudoephedrine.

Like any other supplement or herbal medication it is important to tell your doctor if you are taking it, particularly if you are on any other prescribed or over-the-counter medication. Taking St John's wort at the same time as other antidepressant medication is dangerous and can cause a very serious and potentially fatal condition called serotonin syndrome. If you are thinking about taking St John's wort, have a good chat with your family doctor or pharmacist, who will be able to advise you appropriately.

A Test for Depression

The table on the next page shows a questionnaire used by doctors to help diagnose depression. Known as the PHQ-9, it was developed by Drs Robert L. Spitzer, Janet B.W. Williams, Kurt Kroenke and colleagues, with an educational grant from Pfizer Inc.

Depression

Patient Health Questionnaire – 9 (Depression)

Over the last 2 weeks, how often have you been bothered by any of the following problems?	Not at all	Several days	More than half the days	Nearly every day
1. Little interest or pleasure in doing things	0	1	2	3
2. Feeling down, depressed or hopeless	0	1	2	3
3. Trouble falling or staying asleep, or sleeping too much	0	1	2	3
4. Feeling tired or having little energy	0	1	2	3
5. Poor appetite or overeating	0	1	2	3
6. Feeling bad about yourself – or that you are a failure or have let yourself or your family down	0	1	2	3
7. Trouble concentrating on things, such as reading the newspaper or watching television	0	1	2	3
8. Moving or speaking so slowly that other people could have noticed? Or the opposite – being so fidgety or restless that you have been moving around a lot more than usual	0	1	2	3
9. Thoughts that you would be better off dead or of hurting yourself in some way	0	1	2	3

How Did You Fare?

Depression Severity:

0–4	None
5–9	Mild depression
10–14	Moderate depression
15–19	Moderately severe depression
20–27	Severe depression

Issues to Consider With Your Doctor

Take the time to discuss your ideas, concerns and worries with your doctor. For some men this may be the only sounding board they have to discuss such emotional feelings:

- Could my symptoms indicate depression?
- Is medication the best option for treating my depression?
- What non-drug treatments might help my depression?
- What self-help strategies might help reduce my depression?
- If I decide to take medication, should I pursue talking therapy or counselling as well?

What About Seasonal Affective Disorder (SAD)?

SAD syndrome, also known as 'winter blues', is very common; it is thought to affect at least one in ten Irish men. Maybe the other nine out of ten are in denial! It is not clear exactly what causes it but a lack of sunlight appears to trigger changes in the balance of certain chemicals in the brain, which can trigger a depression-like illness. Symptoms of seasonal affective disorder include:

- Fatigue
- Excess sleep
- Food cravings and weight gain
- Feeling a little 'blue'

- Sometimes some of the other symptoms of depression (as described above)

My own personal observation is that these symptoms become especially noticeable in the post-Christmas months of January and February.

What Are the Treatment Options for SAD?

Treatment options include the standard treatment options for other types of depression, including St John's wort or other antidepressant medications. A good exercise programme can be protective and a bit of winter sun can work wonders. Light therapy can also be an effective option for some men.

Light Therapy for SAD

Light therapy can be an effective way to help winter blues by stimulating the brain chemicals that help mood. This treatment consists of sitting in front of a very bright light of about 2500 watts (about ten times the strength of an ordinary light bulb) for about half an hour every day. The light must face you, but you do not have to look directly into it. So, you can continue to work, read and so on while facing the light source.

Light therapy appears to be safe. The light boxes used to treat SAD do not emit much ultraviolet light, so sunburn is not a problem; however, some people do complain of headaches and irritability. Tanning machines are not a suitable source of light to treat SAD as they cause sunburn.

Treatment is best started in the autumn, when symptoms begin, and continued until the spring. Some people find it beneficial to use it first thing in the morning as an alarm clock, whereby the light comes on 40 minutes before their normal wakening time. This has been described as a 'natural dawn'.

People can notice an improvement in several days, but it can take several weeks for symptoms to improve.

What About Natural Sunlight?

Natural sunlight, even on an overcast wintery day, can help your mood. Certainly, if you have the opportunity to get outdoors for an hour, this can be helpful. However, for many indoor office workers, this is just not possible, particularly in the cold wet climate of the Irish winter.

Suicide

Here in Ireland over 450 people committed suicide last year. Men outnumber women by a ratio of four to one in terms of death by suicide. Suicide is a leading cause of death in young people.

Risk Factors for Suicide

Suicide is often a tragic consequence of undiagnosed or untreated depression, and may occur in the context of alcohol or drug abuse. Other common risk factors for suicide in men can include chronic pain, major stress – including traumatic life events and recent loss – social isolation and loneliness. Depression in particular can play a large role in suicide. The teenage years can be emotionally volatile and issues relating to self-esteem, body image and lack of confidence can be very real ones for teenagers. Depression is a real issue of concern for teenagers and can also be a major risk factor for teen suicide.

Suicide in Elderly Men

The highest suicide rates of any age group occur among men aged over 65 years. Depression in elderly men that is undiagnosed and so untreated is a major risk factor. Others include major life events such as retirement, loss of independence, bereavement and isolation or loneliness. Chronic ill health, including chronic pain or disability, can also be factors.

Antidepressants and Suicide

Sometimes depression medication can cause an increase – rather than a decrease – in depression and suicidal thoughts and feelings. Therefore, anyone on antidepressants should be aware of and watch out for increases in suicidal thoughts and behaviours. This is thought to be most important early on in the treatment programme and when the dose of medication is changed.

Warning Signs of Suicide

- Signs of severe depression:
  o unrelenting low mood
  o pessimism
  o hopelessness
  o worthlessness
- Social withdrawal
  o Sleep problems
  o Increased alcohol and/or other drug use
  o Impulsive behaviour and taking unnecessary risks
  o Talking about suicide or expressing a strong wish to die
  o Unexpected mood swings, including rage or anger

Take any suicidal talk or behaviour seriously as it is often a cry for help. More subtle warning signs of suicide are feelings of hopelessness or worthlessness. People who feel hopeless about their situation may talk about 'unbearable' feelings, predict a bleak future and state that they have nothing to look forward to. A suicidal person may have dramatic mood swings or sudden personality changes, such as becoming very withdrawn, losing interest in day-to-day activities, neglecting his appearance and showing big changes in eating or sleeping habits.

Although most depressed people are not suicidal, most suicidal people are depressed. Serious depression can be manifested in obvious sadness, but often it is expressed as a loss of pleasure or withdrawal from activities that had been enjoyable. One can help prevent suicide through early recognition and treatment of depression and other mental illnesses.

Some Misconceptions About Suicide

• Men who commit suicide are unwilling to seek help. FALSE:

Many suicide victims have sought medical help within the six months prior to their deaths.

• People who talk about suicide won't really commit suicide. FALSE:

Many men who attempt or commit suicide give some warning clue in advance. It may be something that's said; statements like 'I'd be better off dead' or 'I can't see any way out' should raise the alarm. Rather than ignoring talk about suicide, discussing the subject openly can be helpful.

• If a man is determined to commit suicide nothing is going to stop him. FALSE:

The sense of hopelessness that can be experienced with severe depression can lead to impulsive thoughts of suicide and temporarily push someone over the edge.

Prevention of Suicide

Suicide prevention starts with recognising the warning signs and taking them seriously. If you think a friend or family member is considering suicide, don't be afraid to bring up the subject. Be willing to listen. Speak up if you're concerned and encourage the person to seek professional support from a doctor.

- Take it seriously:

Many people who commit suicide give some warning of their intentions to a friend or family member. Therefore all suicide threats and attempts should be taken seriously.

- Be willing to listen:

Be a good listener and let a suicidal person express his feelings. Provide understanding, reassurance and support. Let him know you care.

- Get appropriate help:

Get the person appropriate professional help as soon as possible. If necessary, bring him to his doctor. You can make a difference.

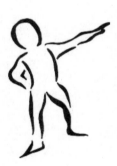

Key Points

- Depression is common and often goes undiagnosed and untreated in Irish men.
- Anyone can get depression and it does not mean you are weak or in any way inadequate.
- Being aware of the symptoms of depression can help you to take action and seek help from your GP.

- Depression can usually be effectively treated with lifestyle changes, counselling and medication, either alone or in combination.
- Medication for depression is not addictive.
- Suicide remains a major cause of death in Irish men.
- Your mental health is every bit as important as your physical health. Look after it!

16

Common and Embarrassing
Men's Health Problems

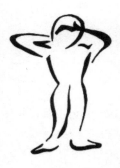

There are a number of common health issues that men can find embarrassing. These types of issues are likely to be suffered in silence or ignored by men. Occasionally they are brought up at the end of the consultation: 'Any cure for piles, doc?' More often though, men suffer in silence, sometimes with nasty consequences. At times as a doctor you are more likely to be confronted with these issues at a hurling match or even the supermarket.

This chapter discusses a number of common men's health problems that men can find embarrassing, and also a number of conditions which, while not embarrassing, are certainly common in men.

Piles (Haemorrhoids)

Piles are small blood-filled swellings of the veins of the back passage area (lower rectum and anus). They are very common and affect up to 50 per cent of men at some stage. They may be present for years and cause no symptoms until bleeding occurs. They may be located at the beginning of the anal canal (internal piles) or at the anal opening (external piles). Piles are not dangerous.

What Causes Piles?

Anything that increases the pressure in the back passage area can cause piles. Constipation and straining at the toilet during bowel movements may cause piles by increasing the pressure in the anal or rectal veins. Other factors include cigarette smoking, a low-fibre diet, heavy lifting, prolonged sitting or standing, obesity, anal intercourse, and loss of muscle tone due to old age or rectal surgery. A family history of piles also plays an important role.

What Are the Symptoms of Piles?

Symptoms can vary depending on the severity or extent of the piles and can include the following:

- Itchy bottom
- Mucus discharge following a bowel movement
- Bleeding from the back passage – this tends to be bright red in colour and can vary from bright red stained blood on the toilet paper to blood dripping into the toilet bowl after a bowel movement. This blood is not mixed with the stool.
- A sensation of rectal fullness may occur or a feeling that the bowel has not emptied fully after a bowel motion (if you have large piles)
- Soiling of faeces can be seen with severe cases of piles.

Piles are usually not painful unless they get blocked over or 'thrombosed', in which case they can be very painful.

If I Think I Have Symptoms of Piles, What Should I Do?

If you think you have symptoms that could indicate piles the best thing to do is have yourself checked out by your GP. By taking a history and conducting an examination your GP will be able to determine the best course of action, including the necessity or otherwise of further investigations.

Rapid assessment is essential if you have bleeding and/or a change in bowel habit as these symptoms may indicate early colorectal cancer, which is a potentially curable condition if caught early.

What Is a Perianal Hematoma?

This is an external pile, where a small bump is found on the outside part of the anus. It often has no symptoms, but if a blood clot forms inside it, it can become extremely painful and bleed for a few days. Eventually it shrinks away, forming a small skin tag.

Treatment of Piles

Piles can often be treated by simple measures like a high-fibre diet and plenty of fluids. Laxative drugs may be prescribed to prevent constipation and soften the stools. There are various creams, ointments and suppositories available to help the symptoms of piles. Preparations containing a steroid can help with swelling or inflammation while preparations containing an anaesthetic can help with pain. These preparations should only be used when they are clinically indicated and for not longer than five to seven days at a stretch. Sometimes these topical anaesthetic creams can sensitise the skin around the anus and actually cause an itchy bottom.

More troublesome piles may require specialist referral to a surgeon. There are several treatment options, including banding. This is a procedure with a high success rate where a rubber band is placed at the bottom of the pile, cutting off its blood supply and causing the pile to 'die' and fall off after a few days. Other options include injecting the piles, causing them to shrivel, and in some cases the pile can be removed surgically under general anaesthetic.

How Can Piles Be Prevented?

Prevention is better than cure and this applies to piles also. Keeping the bowel motions regular and soft, thereby avoiding constipation and straining on the toilet, is the key. The following will help in this regard:

- Drink plenty of fluids, enough each day to keep your urine clear. This will suggest that you are well hydrated. Adults should aim to drink about 2 litres per day (about 3.5 pints).
- Eat plenty of fibre in the diet, including fresh fruit and vegetables and wholegrain bread. Consider fibre supplements.
- Develop and maintain good toileting habits.
- Avoid delaying or putting off going to the toilet when you have the need to go. The longer you delay, the more fluid can be potentially absorbed out of the stool, making it harder to pass when you eventually go.
- Avoid straining at the toilet.
- Be careful with the use of medications, including over-the-counter medicines. For example, codeine is a common cause of constipation and is found in over-the-counter medications such as Solpadeine and Nurofen Plus.

Itchy Bottom

Many men who suffer from the symptoms of an itchy bottom feel embarrassed and are reluctant to seek medical advice. Itchy bottom is a common problem for men. The condition is known medically as *pruritus ani.* The underlying causes are rarely serious and treatment is usually highly successful. Symptoms include an ongoing chronic feeling of itchiness around the back passage area. The sensation of itching is often worse after going to the toilet or just before sleep at bedtime. However it can occur at any time. It can be aggravated by stress, anxiety, heat, moisture or various allergies.

What Are the Causes?

Sometimes the cause of *pruritus ani* is never found. However, there are many recognised causes. These include the following:

- Fungal infections such as thrush, which tend to thrive in warm moist environments
- Thread worm infection, which is a common cause of itching in children. Children can pass this infection on quite easily to adults in the same home. This is why hand-washing after going to the toilet and short clean fingernails are essential.
- Skin conditions such as eczema or psoriasis
- Dermatitis of the anal skin is also a common cause of itching. This is often caused by a reaction to sweat, moisture or small amounts of faecal material around the anal area.
- A reaction to different irritants, including soaps, coloured toilet paper and sometimes the ingredients in creams and ointments used to treat piles.
- Haemorrhoids or piles
- Other infections, including warts, sexually transmitted infections and scabies, can cause an itch around the back passage. There will often be other associated symptoms of these infections.
- An anal fissure, which is a localised crack in the anal skin, can cause itchiness around the back passage, often associated with pain or discomfort.

- Allergies to various foodstuffs not properly digested can cause localised irritation and itchiness around the back passage. Examples of these food stuffs include citrus fruits, tomatoes and sometimes drinking large amounts of alcohol, beer or coffee.
- Medication should be considered as a potential cause of any symptom and *pruritus ani* is no exception. In this case particularly, laxatives and some antibiotics may be the underlying cause.
- Rarer causes of an itchy bottom will include some medical conditions that can cause generalised itch around the body. These may include anaemia, lymphoma and kidney failure. Rarely a tumour of the anus or rectum can cause an itch.

It is important to remember that if you have symptoms such as bleeding, altered bowel habit – including persistent constipation or diarrhoea or a mixture of both – mucus discharge or lumps around the back passage then you need to see your doctor quickly. This will allow for any potential bowel cancer to be promptly diagnosed and treatment started.

What Should I Do If I Have Symptoms of Pruritus Ani?

The best thing to do is see your GP and have these symptoms evaluated medically, especially if the itch is troublesome or persistent and definitely if it is associated with any other worrying symptoms as described above.

The treatment will depend on the underlying cause. For example, piles or an anal fissure may need specific surgical treatment, thrush may respond very well to antifungal creams, threadworms to specific worm medication and so on. If there is evidence of inflammation, eczema or dermatitis around the anal area then a short course of a steroid cream may help.

There are also several specific self-help measures that can help stop itchy bottom:

- Scrupulous hygiene around the anus – bath or shower daily and wash the anal area with clear water only. Avoid soap or, if using soap, only use bland non-scented soap such as emulsifying ointment. Wash the anal area after going to the toilet, so as to clear any remnants of faeces, which could potentially irritate the skin. Consider moist tissues such as baby wipes to clean the anal area.
- Keep the anal area dry – after washing pat the area gently, rather than rubbing, with a soft towel. Wear loose cotton underwear and avoid tight-fitting trousers. Avoid excess heat and try to avoid excess sweating. If this is not possible, consider putting some clear tissue in your underwear to absorb the excess moisture.
- After toileting consider applying some emulsifying ointment topically to the anal area. This can act as a very effective barrier and prevent irritation of the anal skin by sweat or moisture.
- Avoid potential irritants – use plain uncoloured toilet paper, wipe and clean gently after passing faeces, and avoid deodorants, scented soap, bubble bath, etc.
- Consider whether anything in your diet is playing a role in your condition. Keep a food diary. Try to eliminate one foodstuff at a time, particularly those that are known to be associated with anal itch and irritation, such as beer, tea, coffee, citrus fruits and tomatoes. Remember that tomatoes are invaluable for your prostate and that fresh fruit is full of antioxidants so it is important that these excellent foodstuffs do not get blamed inappropriately.
- Minimise your scratching. This is because scratching an itchy part of the skin tends to cause that area of the skin to get itchier, which in turn causes you to scratch more. This causes a scratch–itch cycle that can lead to very irritated itchy skin. Sometimes

295

people with *pruritus ani* will scratch during their sleep. Therefore, make sure sensible precautions are followed, including keeping your fingernails short and clean and even wearing cotton gloves at night if necessary.

Medical Options

Sometimes doctors will prescribe a steroid cream to be used topically for a few days to settle down any inflamed areas. These do not work on infected skin, which requires an antibiotic. Antihistamine medication taken at night-time may have some benefit in reducing the sensation of itch in the skin. In more persistent cases you may need to be referred to a skin specialist for specialised testing, including skin patch testing.

Bad Breath

Bad breath, known medically as halitosis (pronounced hal-it-oas-is), is common and embarrassing for many men. The best way to know if you have bad breath is to ask your partner or a close friend.

What Causes Bad Breath?

There are many varied causes of bad breath. Gum disease and poor oral hygiene are common causes of bad breath. Naturally it is important to brush your teeth regularly. However, even regular brushing of your teeth may not prevent gum disease. Symptoms of gum disease include bad breath and gums that bleed easily when brushing. Gum disease is usually painless but if the gums become acutely infected and swollen then the gums can become painful as well. Gum disease is caused by plaque, which is a sticky bacteria that forms on the teeth everyday and can lodge between the teeth in the area where the teeth meets the gums. This plaque eventually causes a foul stale odour. Regular flossing of your teeth has an important role to play in keeping plaque levels down.

Sinus problems or allergies often cause a post nasal drip, where mucus runs from the back of the nose down into the mouth. This can cause bacteria and bugs to accumulate on the back of the tongue, which can cause bad breath.

Foods commonly associated with bad breath include:

- Spicy foods such as curries
- Garlic
- Some vegetables, including onions, cabbage and broccoli
- Smoked foods such as smoked mackerel
- Processed meats such as salami, which is high in nitrates
- Fizzy drinks

These foods are a common cause of bad breath for two reasons. Firstly, the odour from some foodstuffs can remain in the mouth. Secondly, some of these foods release gases as they are broken down in the stomach. This gas can come back up to the mouth and contribute to bad breath. Similarly, alcohol can also cause bad breath.

Any condition that causes drying of the mouth can lead to bad breath. This is often why we have bad breath first thing in the morning, which is almost universal because when we are sleeping we do not produce saliva, which helps keep the mouth clean. Smoking also causes bad breath by reducing the flow of saliva; this is known as 'smokers' breath'. Dry mouth can also be caused by other medical conditions such as heartburn and belching or by medication, particularly drugs that are used to treat depression and bladder disorders.

Not eating regular meals can cause bad breath. When we are hungry our bodies start to break down fat. Ketones – a by-product of fat breakdown – are exhaled in the breath and can cause bad breath.

How Do I Treat Bad Breath?

Obviously being aware of it and being aware of the potential causes listed above is the first step. The following steps will also help:

- If you smoke, stop! This is the single biggest gift you can give your health in the long term.
- Go for a proper dental check-up.
- Make sure you know how to brush and floss your teeth properly. Regular flossing and using a tooth pick after meals can make a big difference. Use a tongue cleaner to brush the back of the tongue, thereby clearing it of bacteria.
- Keep a detailed food and liquid diary for a week or so, including a weekend. This will allow you to reflect accurately on your dietary habits.
- Make sure you are not skipping meals, particularly breakfast.
- Make sure you are drinking enough fluids (at least 2 litres per day) to stay adequately hydrated. Keeping an eye on your urine and making sure it is pale or clear is a helpful indicator.
- Eat plenty of fresh fruit. Pineapple appears to be particularly good as it contains an enzyme that helps clear the mouth of bacteria.
- Drinking black tea can help some people with bad breath as it helps clear the mouth of harmful bacteria. Various green and herbal teas can also be good for bad breath, particularly camomile and peppermint.
- Eating parsley seems to help with bad breath.
- Get any associated medical conditions such as heartburn or sinusitis properly assessed and treated.
- If you suffer from dry mouth, get this assessed by your doctor.
- Chewing sugar-free gum helps the production of saliva, which can be helpful in clearing particles of food from the mouth.

Using a mouthwash can also help disguise bad breath. Some mouthwashes contain antibacterial properties and they tend to be most effective if they are used at night before bedtime. However, some mouthwashes are acidic, which can potentially damage tooth enamel, and others can temporarily stain and darken teeth. While mouthwashes can be a very useful part of an integrated approach to the problem of bad breath, they are not a cure. It is much better to determine what the underlying causes are and treat those properly rather than just blindly using a mouthwash as a sticking plaster solution.

Finally, there is some evidence now that gum disease may be associated with heart disease. So looking after your oral health and teeth may not be good just for your breath, it may help your heart as well!

Jock Itch

Jock itch, sometimes known as sweat rash, is an itchy rash that occurs on the scrotum and groin area of men. It is caused by a fungus or yeast infection known as *tinea cruris*. Fungi such as *tinea cruris* tend to grow and thrive in warm moist areas. It is a common but underreported condition, as men are often shy or embarrassed about presenting with these types of problems unless they become very bothersome.

What Are the Symptoms?

The symptom of jock itch is usually itching associated with a red rash. This rash often has a little bit of scaling around the edges, and occurs in the groin and scrotum areas. It is commonly seen in sports people because the associated body heat and sweating provides an ideal medium for fungus infections to grow and thrive. It is also common in men who are overweight or obese.

How Is It Treated?

This condition is usually effectively treated by applying an antifungal cream topically twice daily for a couple of weeks. In more severe cases antifungal medication can be taken orally. It is important to try to minimise scratching as this can lead to bacterial infection of the skin, which may need treatment with antibiotics. In this regard keeping the fingernails short and clean is essential. As a condition it is not contagious and it is fine to continue with all athletic activities. It is also helpful to wear cotton underwear and avoid tight-fitting trousers so that the area can breathe.

What Can I Do to Avoid Getting It?

- Wear cotton underwear.
- Avoid tight-fitting trousers.
- Make sure to dry yourself carefully after a shower or bath, particularly in the groin area and around the testicles.
- If you are overweight (BMI greater than 25) then lose weight.
- Be aware of the fact that fungi can thrive in damaged skin. So take care with soaps and shampoos that can potentially irritate the skin. Non-perfumed soaps are best.

Athlete's Foot

This is a yeast or fungus infection that affects the feet. Again it is very common, particularly in feet that are warm and sweaty.

What Are the Symptoms?

Athlete's foot often presents with foot odour. It can also cause itching, classically between the fourth and fifth toes, with the space between these toes being red and scaly. As the infection spreads it can cause itching and scaling on other areas of the foot. Anybody can get athlete's foot but it is particularly common in people who play sport, who suffer from sweaty feet or who spend large amounts of time wearing plastic shoes or runners, which can cause the feet to get warm and sweaty.

Sometimes the infection can spread and involve the nails of the feet. This can result in discoloration of the nail, which can look yellowish, brownish or green, with the nail becoming thickened and sometimes more crumbly in appearance.

The diagnosis of a fungal nail infection can be confirmed by getting your doctor to send a nail clipping to the laboratory to have it analysed for the presence of fungus.

Treatment

Athlete's foot usually responds quite well to the use of antifungal creams. The foot must also be allowed to 'breathe' as much as possible by avoiding wearing runners and tight shoes and by wearing flip flops in the evenings. Fungal nail infection, when confirmed, generally requires treatment with antifungal medication for at least three months.

Snoring and Sleep Apnoea

Snoring is basically caused by wind turbulence when you are breathing in through either your nose or mouth. It occurs when air flows past relaxed tissues in your throat, causing the tissues to vibrate as you breathe and creating hoarse or harsh sounds. As you doze off and progress from a lighter sleep to a deep sleep, the muscles in the roof of your mouth (soft palate), tongue and throat relax. The tissues in your throat can relax enough that they vibrate and may partially obstruct your airway. The narrower your airway, the more forceful the airflow becomes. Tissue vibration increases and your snoring grows louder. Snoring may be an occasional problem or it may be habitual. Snoring is common, especially in men; about half of all men snore at some stage and about 25 per cent of men snore regularly.

The main health consequence of snoring is disturbed sleep of the spouse and/or household and it is a recognised cause of marital disharmony. However, snoring can also be a serious health issue for men.

Sleep Apnoea Syndrome

Sleep apnoea syndrome is a potentially serious condition that is seen in some men who snore. This is where the throat tissues block the airway and prevent you from breathing momentarily. When this happens the blood oxygen level falls and carbon dioxide level rises, which causes arousal, making the person suddenly snort or grunt, heralding the return of breathing. Sleep apnoea syndrome is characterised by these spells of loud snoring followed by episodes of silence. The problem is that this mechanism prevents somebody from getting deep refreshing sleep and they suffer from the clinical effects of sleep deprivation, including daytime drowsiness or sleepiness, poor concentration, headaches and irritability. In addition, sleep apnoea syndrome has adverse effects on the heart and blood pressure, leading to an increased risk of heart arrhythmia, heart attack and stroke.

Clues to Sleep Apnoea

Nearly all men who suffer from sleep apnoea syndrome are snorers; however many snorers do not have sleep apnoea syndrome. Feeling tired, drowsy or sleepy during the day is a major clue to the existence of sleep apnoea syndrome. Ask your spouse or partner if there are any periods during snoring when your breathing tapers off or stops, with silence for a few seconds or more, followed by a grunt or a gasp.

The presence of this is highly suggestive of sleep apnoea syndrome. Other symptoms include poor concentration, irritability and reduced daytime performance. Sleep deprivation can also produce a whole range of other symptoms, from sexual dysfunction to sleep walking.

What Contributes to Snoring?

A variety of factors can lead to snoring, including:

- Cigarette smoking
- Your mouth anatomy – a low, thick, soft palate and enlarged tonsils or tissues in the back of your throat (adenoids) can narrow your airway. Likewise, if the triangular piece of tissue hanging from the soft palate (uvula) is elongated, airflow can be obstructed and vibration increased.
- Being overweight or obese
- Alcohol consumption – snoring can also be brought on by consuming too much alcohol before bedtime. Alcohol relaxes the throat muscles and decreases your natural defences against airway obstruction.
- Upper airway problems such as nasal polyps, nasal blockage or congestion, a crooked partition between your nostrils (deviated nasal septum) or a floppy palate

Other known risk factors include allergies, using sedative drugs and rare conditions, including an overactive thyroid gland.

Tips to Prevent or Reduce Snoring

Appropriate lifestyle changes are important in the treatment of snoring and sleep apnoea syndrome:

- If you smoke, stop.

- Keep your weight healthy. Excess weight is a common risk factor for snoring. Keep your body mass index within the range of 20–25.
- Sleep on your side: lying on your back allows your tongue to fall backward into your throat, which can partially obstruct airflow and cause snoring. Some men find sewing a tennis ball onto the back of their pyjamas can help stop them sleeping on their back.
- Adhesive nasal strips applied to your nose can help increase the size of the nasal passage and help the breathing.
- Get medical assessment and treatment for nasal congestion or obstruction. Problems with nasal allergies or obstruction are a common cause of snoring as a blocked nose means you have to breathe through the mouth, which brings an increased risk of snoring. To correct a deviated septum you may need surgery. Restrict your alcohol intake and avoid sedatives, including sleeping tablets.

Diagnosis

If you snore you should consult your doctor, especially if you have symptoms of sleep apnoea. A diagnosis of sleep apnoea syndrome is confirmed by a specialist in the area who will perform sleep studies, which requires you to spend a night in a specially designed sleep lab that measures the amount of oxygen in your blood during the night, amongst other parameters. Other causes of snoring, including nasal obstruction, may benefit from an opinion from an ENT (ear, nose and throat) specialist.

Treatment Options

If lifestyle changes don't sort out the snoring problem other options can be considered. Mouthpieces that help advance the position of your tongue and soft palate to keep your air passage open can be used. Surgical options include tightening the loose tissues in the back of the throat. Laser surgery on the soft palate can now also be an option in some cases.

The treatment of sleep apnoea syndrome has been revolutionised by the delivery of continuous positive airway pressure (CPAP). This delivers air continuously through your airway while you are sleeping. The most common form of CPAP involves wearing nasal prongs or a pressurised mask on the nose while you are sleeping. The mask is attached to a small pump that forces air through the airway, keeping it open. CPAP is extremely effective and can prevent all complications of sleep apnoea syndrome. However, like many medications or medical devices, it is only as good as the willingness or ability of the person to use it regularly.

Haemochromatosis – The Celtic Storage Disease

Iron is a valuable mineral that helps make the blood rich in oxygen, helps the blood to carry oxygen to the muscles and also helps the brain and immune systems. However, while a certain amount of iron is good for us, more certainly isn't better. Haemochromatosis is an inherited condition in which the body tends to absorb too much iron so that iron leaks out of the blood and into the joints and body organs such as the liver, heart and pancreas. This excess iron can damage the normal functioning of these organs.

Until a few years ago haemochromatosis was thought to be a fairly rare condition. Now we know it as one of the most common inherited disorders. Up to one in every five Irish men may be carriers of the gene for this condition. Men are five times more likely than women to develop iron overload, and they usually experience symptoms at an earlier age. Women tend to store less iron than men as they lose it through menstruation and pregnancy.

What Are the Symptoms?

Haemochromatosis generally causes no symptoms before the age of 30 in men. Even then it can be a silent condition for many years. However, eventually when the iron leaks out of the blood and into the organs around the body, symptoms will start to occur. These symptoms are varied and may include the following:

- Diabetes
- Joint problems (arthritis) – any joint in the body can be affected
- Stomach pains
- Weakness, tiredness and chronic fatigue
- Erectile dysfunction, loss of sex drive or difficulty with erections
- Mood swings, irritability, depression or memory difficulties
- A permanent tan or bronzing of the skin
- Cardiomyopathy – where the heart muscle does not pump as efficiently as it should, leading to heart irregularities and heart failure
- Liver problems – swelling and inflammation, abnormal liver blood tests and eventually cirrhosis or liver cancer

How Is this Condition Inherited?

We all have about 30,000 genes in our bodies, which are tiny information and control centres in the cells of the body that control how the body works and grows. A mutation in just one gene can drastically alter the way your body works. To inherit haemochromatosis you need to inherit a defective gene from both of your parents. Therefore it is not necessary for either of your parents to have had haemochromatosis for you to get the condition. If you simply inherit the gene from one parent then you will be a carrier; this means you are not likely to develop haemochromatosis yourself, but you can pass on this defective gene to your own children. If you inherit the gene from both parents you will develop the condition yourself.

Relatives of patients with haemochromatosis should be tested to see if they are carrying the defective gene. This includes brothers, sisters, parents, partners and children from the age of 18 years upwards.

What Tests Can Be Done To Diagnose Haemochromatosis?

Iron overload can be detected with two blood tests even if there are no symptoms:

- Serum transferrin saturation: this test measures the amount of iron bound to a protein (transferrin) that carries iron in your blood. Transferrin saturation values greater than 50 per cent are considered too high.
- Serum ferritin: this test measures the amount of iron stored in your body. Figures over 300 are considered too high. Other infectious and inflammatory conditions can also cause elevated ferritin.

Genetic testing can be carried out by taking a blood test to see if you have the genes for haemochromatosis.

Remember, knowledge is power; by being aware of the possible symptoms of haemochromatosis you can raise this possibility with your own doctor if you have concerns.

How Is This Condition Treated?

Treatment for haemochromatosis is incredibly simple: it involves regularly removing blood, just as if you were donating it. Removing a pint of blood from the body removes about a quarter of a gram of iron. The frequency of blood letting required varies from person to person. Some people need to have this procedure carried out at weekly intervals. For others, monthly or less frequently will suffice. The target with treatment is to get the serum ferritin level below fifty. This treatment can be very effective at bringing the amount of iron in the body down. However, it cannot reverse complications of haemochromatosis such as cirrhosis or diabetes. Therefore, early detection is better than cure. The goal with haemochromatosis is to detect it at an early stage before the complications have set in. Medical professionals are increasingly aware of this important condition, particularly as it is now recognised as being so common. The challenge, as with all things relating to health, is for men to educate themselves about these conditions so they can then make appropriate health choices.

What About a Low-Iron Diet?

Unfortunately dietary changes are really of no benefit in haemochromatosis. This is because a normal diet contains about ten times as much iron as we need, so normally only 10 per cent of the iron that we eat is absorbed into our body. However, the following dietary suggestions are recommended:

- Tea, coffee and brown bread contain phytates, which are vitamins that can help reduce iron absorption.
- Avoid all vitamins, supplements or tonics containing iron.
- Avoid large doses of Vitamin C, as it enhances iron absorption and may also make it easier for iron to be deposited in organs around the body.
- Minimise your intake of iron-rich foods such as red meat and offal (kidneys, liver, etc.), and breads or cereals heavily fortified with iron.
- Avoid alcohol – alcohol and iron combine to cause more liver damage.

Coeliac Disease

Coeliac disease is a genetic bowel disorder caused by an allergy to gluten, a protein that is found in wheat, rye and barley. Most people with coeliac disease can eat oats, although some people with a more severe sensitivity to gluten cannot.

How Common Is It and What Are the Symptoms?

Coeliac disease affects about 3 per cent of the Irish population. It can present in early childhood with frequent smelly stools, lack of growth, anaemia, failure to thrive and weight loss. However, in many adults the condition is not diagnosed until middle age and people often present with very vague and non-specific bowel or stomach complaints such as wind, gas, constipation, bloating and sometimes pale smelly stools that are difficult to flush. Coeliac disease may also be a cause of tiredness, including chronic fatigue.

How Is the Condition Diagnosed?

Blood tests may show anaemia, which can be due to a combination of a lack of iron and a lack of folic acid. Specific coeliac blood tests can check for the presence of antigluten and other antibodies. The diagnosis is confirmed by carrying out biopsies of a part of the bowel known as the jejunum. This test will be carried out by a hospital specialist.

How Is Coeliac Disease Treated?

The cornerstone of the management of coeliac disease is simply to avoid gluten and to strictly follow a gluten-free diet. This means no wheat, no barley and no rye, and avoiding any food containing these ingredients, including bread, cakes and pies. Gluten-free biscuits, flour, bread and pasta are available. Rice, maize, soy, potatoes, sugar, jam, syrup and treacle are allowed, along with moderate quantities of oats. People with coeliac disease are at risk of developing several complications; this is largely due to a lack of compliance with a gluten-free diet. Human nature and a dislike of restrictions mean that people may be inclined to not follow medical advice when they don't feel sick. However, sufferers who do not comply properly with a strict gluten-free diet have an increased risk of osteoporosis and of both iron and folate deficiency anaemias. There is some evidence that patients with coeliac disease are at increased risk of some bowel cancers, including one known as intestinal lymphoma. It is thought that adherence to a strict gluten-free diet decreases this risk.

Gout

Gout can be an extremely painful condition that mainly affects men. In fact gout is the most common cause of pain, redness and tenderness (painful arthritis) in men over the age of 40. Gout is caused by a build-up in the body of a chemical called uric acid.

What Is Uric Acid?

Uric acid is naturally produced by the body as a result of the breakdown of purines as part of the body's normal ongoing daily wear, tear and repair process. Purines are substances found in all of the body's cells, and in many foods. This is a normal and healthy process. Uric acid from this process is generally cleared by the kidneys. Imagine the kidneys as being like a sieve which filters all the bad stuff from the body, keeping the good stuff in. With gout the kidneys become less efficient at filtering (the holes in the sieve become smaller) so more uric acid is retained in the body. This is what happens when you drink alcohol and is why many heavy drinkers get gout. When the uric acid reaches a certain level it can then escape into the bloodstream and enter the joints, causing pain.

Some people can just produce too much uric acid (one reason why some men who don't drink alcohol can still get gout). Uric acid can also be found in our diets, particularly in purine-rich foods like red meat (especially offal), duck, seafood (especially sardines and anchovies), gravy, kidney beans, peas and lentils. Other culprits can include shellfish, spinach, asparagus, cauliflower, mushrooms, beer and other forms of alcohol.

Binge drinking and extreme fasting can also cause uric acid levels to rise, as can certain medications, such as thiazide diuretics and niacin (Vitamin B_3), which is often taken to boost HDL (good) cholesterol (see Chapter 6). Sometimes there are genetic factors involved that cause the uric acid level to be too high.

It is the build-up of high uric acid over a long period of time that tends to cause gout. The higher the uric acid level the higher the chance of developing gout. When uric acid leaks out of the blood it enters the joints, most commonly the big toe. Occasionally it can affect other joints, including the hands. The attack usually comes on suddenly, causing pain, and within a few hours the affected joint can become red, hot, swollen and painful.

Diagnosis of Gout

The diagnosis of gout is often straightforward. Certainly any man who has suffered recurring attacks of gout will know immediately when they have been struck down by it. However, sometimes other forms of arthritis or infection can mimic gout. A high uric acid level supports the diagnosis of gout, but it is not as black and white as it seems: some people can have a high uric acid level for many years without developing gout. If the diagnosis is uncertain the doctor may remove a small amount of fluid from the joint; the presence of uric acid crystals in the joint fluid confirms the diagnosis beyond doubt.

Complications of Gout

Recurrent attacks of gout can lead to chronic gout, which can cause a form of arthritis in the joints and permanent joint damage. Swellings, called tophi, can occur in the joints due to a build-up of large amounts of uric acid crystals. These uric acid crystals can also deposit in the kidneys, causing kidney stones.

Treatment of Gout

Acute attacks of gout can be effectively treated by taking anti-inflammatory medication. Caution is needed with anti-inflammatories, however, as they can affect the stomach and kidneys. Other options include colchicine (although this can cause vomiting and diarrhoea) or short courses of steroids.

If someone is suffering from recurrent attacks of gout they can be prescribed medication, known as allopurinol, to lower the uric acid level. However, while allopurinol is very effective at preventing attacks of gout, it must be stopped if someone suffers an attack while taking it as it can make an acute episode of gout worse.

Tips to Prevent Gout

Drinking lots of water is important to flush out the kidneys and help to remove uric acid from the body. While only about 10 per cent of uric acid comes from our diet, making some dietary changes can be worthwhile. It is recommended to cut back on purine-rich foods (see page 311) and keep your alcohol consumption within safe limits, particularly avoiding binge drinking. Keep your weight healthy (BMI 20–25). If you are overweight this puts extra strain and pressure on your joints as well as increasing the risk of high uric acid levels and gout. Avoid crash diets as they can increase uric acid levels in the blood, and also low-carbohydrate diets that are high in protein and fat, which can increase uric acid levels.

Kidney Stones

Kidney stones are small bits of mineral and acid salts inside the kidneys. They are caused by the urine flowing through the kidneys becoming rich or heavy in minerals that form into crystals, which in time can stick together, solidify and develop into tiny bits of gravel and eventually stones. Normally these substances are diluted in the urine. The main mineral found in most kidney stones is calcium, while others less commonly found include oxalate or phosphate. About 10 per cent of kidney stones are due to excess uric acid.

How Common Are Kidney Stones?

Kidney stones mainly occur in men. An Irish man has about a 10 per cent chance of getting a kidney stone at some stage during his life, most commonly between the ages of 20 and 50. They also have a nasty habit of recurring. Up to 50 per cent of men will suffer a reoccurrence within ten years of getting a kidney stone.

What Are the Symptoms of Kidney Stones?

Sometimes kidney stones can remain dormant, or silent, for years if they occupy a wide part of the ureter (the tube connecting the kidneys and bladder), so you may not even know you have one. If your urine is tested by your doctor at this stage, traces of blood may be detected. However, once the gravel or stone moves into a narrower part of the ureter, blocking it, symptoms develop.

The main symptom of a kidney stone is pain, also known as renal colic. The pain of kidney stones is often very severe. It can start suddenly in the lower back and often radiates around to the groin and down into the testicles or scrotum. The pain can vary in intensity with episodes of severe pain lasting from 20 to 60 minutes. It is usually impossible to get into a comfortable position when you have this pain. The excruciating pain is often associated with:

- Nausea and/or vomiting
- Bloody urine that may be red or brown in colour
- Cloudy or foul-smelling urine
- A persistent urge to urinate, with burning pain
- A high temperature and sometimes shakes or rigors if an infection is present

Kidney stones that don't cause these symptoms may show up on X-rays when you seek medical care for other problems, such as blood in your urine or recurring urinary tract infections.

What Are Kidney Stones Made Of?

Most kidney stones contain crystals of more than one type. However, it can be easier to figure out the underlying cause of the kidney stone if the makeup of the stone is known.

- Calcium stones – almost 80 per cent of kidney stones are calcium stones, usually in the form of calcium oxalate.
- Struvite stones are almost always the result of urinary tract infections. They may become big enough to fill the inside of the kidney and they have a characteristic stag's horn shape.
- Uric acid stones are related to protein and purine metabolism, with high levels of uric acid also causing gout.
- Cystine stones are uncommon and are due to genetic disorders.

Risk Factors for Kidney Stones

Kidney stones usually don't have one single identifiable cause. However, these factors may increase your risk of developing kidney stones:

- Dehydration – if you don't drink enough fluids, especially water, your urine will have higher concentrations of substances that can form stones. It's also important to rehydrate after exercise and when in the heat.

- A family history of kidney stones
- A previous history of kidney stones
- Diet – a high-protein, high-sodium and low-calcium diet can increase your risk of some types of kidney stones.

Other risk factors include high blood pressure, obesity and prolonged immobility, for example, being bed-bound with a broken leg. In addition, any bowel disorder that reduces your ability to absorb calcium will lead to more oxalates in the urine, which can lead to stone formation. These can include gastric bypass surgery, inflammatory bowel disease and chronic diarrhoea.

Tests and Diagnosis

If your doctor suspects you have kidney stones, you're likely to have blood tests to look for excess calcium or uric acid and a 24-hour collection of urine to analyse its content. You may also need a scan of the urinary tract. However, nothing beats hard evidence and if you can recover a stone you have passed, perhaps by peeing through a strainer, then it can be analysed.

Treatment

The treatment of kidney stones depends on the type of stone as well as the underlying cause. Sometimes the stones will pass on their own and drinking large amounts of liquid can help this process. Sometimes larger stones can be treated with lithotripsy, which is a form of ultrasonic shock therapy, causing the stone to break into tiny fragments that are then passed in the urine. Occasionally surgery is needed to remove kidney stones. Kidney stones may remain silent and cause no long-term problems. However, there is the risk of long-term kidney damage as well as kidney infection.

Prevention

Lifestyle changes can prevent kidney stones in many cases. The best way to prevent kidney stones is to drink lots of fluids and avoid dehydration. This means drinking enough fluid to keep the urine pale or clear in colour. Urine that is yellowish in colour means dehydration. For most men this means drinking several extra glasses of water a day on top of their usual fluid intake. If you have already had a kidney stone you will have to drink even more fluid (up to 3 litres a day) to keep the urine very dilute, thereby preventing crystals from forming in the urine. The best fluid to drink is good old-fashioned water. A glass of lemonade made with real lemons is also thought to be good as lemons increase the amount of citrates in the urine, which can help prevent stone formation.

If you have a history of calcium-based kidney stones you should certainly avoid calcium or Vitamin D supplements. However, for many men a low-calcium diet doesn't appear to reduce the chances of getting kidney stones. A diet low in salt and animal protein is thought to be helpful in preventing kidney stones.

It may be advisable to avoid foods with high amounts of oxalate as this is the substance that can bind calcium in the urine, thereby helping to form calcium oxalate stones. Foods that are high in oxalate include rhubarb, parsley, nuts (especially almonds), spinach, beets, instant coffee and chocolate. As with all other dietary recommendations, moderation is the key.

Uric acid stones are a complication of gout. To prevent these you need to keep your uric acid levels low through a combination of high fluid intake and a low-protein diet, staying away from red meat and shellfish in particular.

Osteoporosis

Osteoporosis is a disease that causes the skeleton to weaken and the bones to break. A useful analogy is that of a big thick coffee mug turning into a dainty china cup that eventually cracks and crumbles. It poses a significant threat to many Irish men, as up to one in every five men will be affected by it at some stage. Yet, despite the large number of men affected, osteoporosis in men remains under-diagnosed and under-reported. Many Irish men view osteoporosis solely as a 'woman's disease'. Osteoporosis is called a silent disease because it usually progresses without symptoms until a fracture occurs.

Fractures resulting from osteoporosis most commonly occur in the hip, spine and wrist. Hip fractures are especially dangerous and men can die from their complications or be left permanently disabled.

What Causes Osteoporosis?

Bone is constantly being built up and broken down in the body. Generally, peak bone mass is reached at about the age of 35, which is when our bones are at their strongest. After this age we start to lose more calcium from our bones slowly over time, causing our bones to gradually weaken. In some people the bones become fragile more quickly than in others. Once bones lose a certain amount of calcium they are more likely to break from a fall – this weakening of the bones is known as osteoporosis.

Men in their fifties do not experience the rapid loss of bone mass that women do in the years following menopause. By age 65 or 70, however, men and women are losing bone mass at the same rate, and the absorption of calcium, an essential nutrient for bone health throughout life, decreases in both sexes.

What Are the Symptoms?

Symptoms of osteoporosis in men may include a fracture occurring after a relatively minor trauma, loss of height or sudden back pain (the latter two symptoms caused by a vertebral bone in the back breaking). In many cases there are no symptoms until the later stages. Untreated osteoporosis can lead to progressive pain, loss of height, loss of independence, premature disability and even death.

Risk Factors for Osteoporosis in Men

Several risk factors have been linked to osteoporosis in men:

- Unhealthy lifestyle habits such as smoking, excessive alcohol use, low calcium intake and inadequate physical exercise
- Age – the older you are, the greater your risk
- Use of steroids and other drugs, including drugs to treat epilepsy and anti-cancer drugs
- Lowered testosterone levels
- Chronic chest problems such as emphysema, asthma and cystic fibrosis
- Conditions affecting the gut, like coeliac disease, that prevent absorption of nutrients like calcium, magnesium and Vitamin D
- An overactive thyroid
- Immobilisation
- Some types of arthritis, such as rheumatoid arthritis

Steroids are medications used to treat diseases such as asthma and rheumatoid arthritis. Bone loss is a very common side affect of these medications. Therefore, men taking these medications should talk to their doctor about having a bone mineral density (BMD) test. Abnormally low levels of sex hormones cause osteoporosis in women after the menopause. Similarly, lowered testosterone levels can also cause osteoporosis in men. Immobilisation during illness or after a fracture or surgery can result in significant bone loss. Therefore a good diet and a proactive rehabilitation programme are essential to help counteract this. Even astronauts in space are prone to osteoporosis because they are in a gravity-free environment.

How Is Osteoporosis Diagnosed?

Osteoporosis can be effectively treated if it is detected before significant bone loss has occurred. The gold standard test for osteoporosis is a type of bone mineral density (BMD) test known as a DEXA scan. This test can identify osteoporosis, determine your risk of fractures (broken bones) and measure your response to osteoporosis treatment. It is a painless test, like having an x-ray, but with much less exposure to radiation. It can measure bone density at your hip and spine.

How Can Osteoporosis Be Prevented?

Men should take the following steps to preserve their bone health:

- Avoid smoking.
- Reduce your alcohol intake to less than 21 units per week.
- Increase your level of physical activity, especially weight-bearing exercises like walking, jogging, and racquet or team sports. Lifting weights can also help; the main idea is that both the bones and muscles work against gravity.
- Make sure you get enough calcium and Vitamin D in your diet. Get out in the sunlight daily to help the body manufacture Vitamin D.
- Talk to your doctor about any medications you may be taking that can affect your bones, such as steroids.
- Recognise and seek treatment for any underlying medical conditions that affect bone health.

What Treatments Are Available?

Once a man has been diagnosed with osteoporosis his doctor may prescribe one of several medications available to strengthen the bone density. A healthy lifestyle, including plenty of weight-bearing exercise and calcium and/or Vitamin D supplements can help. If there is an identifiable underlying cause for the osteoporosis, such as testosterone deficiency, a specific treatment plan may address the underlying cause.

There are several drug treatment options available at present. The best known of these is a group of drugs known as bisphosphonates, which can be taken just once weekly. They can help prevent further calcium loss from the bones and sometimes can help strengthen the bone. Side effects can include inflammation of the food pipe and a possible effect on the jaw known as osteonecrosis. There is a lot of research in this area at present and newer treatments will be available in time. Keep informed about developments in this area.

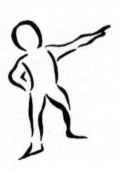

Key Points

- Knowledge is power – stay informed about important men's health issues.
- Don't be embarrassed about seeking help for issues that concern you, even if they are not life-threatening.
- Talk to your doctor; he or she is there to help and advise you.
- Remember: prevention is better than cure.

17

Conclusion – Time to Change for Your Better Health

Irish men can be complex and full of contradictions regarding their health. The facts speak for themselves: Irish men die, on average, at least five years younger then Irish women, often from medical conditions and complications that are preventable. At the moment there is an explosion of diabetes and obesity-related conditions, with complications of heart disease and stroke just around the corner. Irish men have high rates of bowel and prostate cancer, while stress-related illnesses are on the increase.

In the same breath, we know that Irish men are less likely to access healthcare than women. They will often stick their heads in the sand or kid themselves that they are too busy. In my opinion most Irish men do care about their health, but at times there seems to be an 'if it ain't broke don't fix it' mentality. This is the wrong attitude. It is a dangerous assumption to make about your health. Many important health conditions, such as high blood pressure, high cholesterol levels and even diabetes, can remain silent with no symptoms for many years. So you may have health problems for a long time and still feel perfectly well. This is an important point because prevention and early detection are better than cure. If these conditions are detected at an early stage they can be treated and difficult long-term complications can be prevented. We can kid ourselves into thinking that because we feel fine our health must also be fine.

While feeling well is a great place to be at and a good start to better health, it should compliment rather then replace the need for a sensible approach to your long-term health plan. To a large extent your future health is in your own hands. Develop good health habits now and they can gift you a lifetime of better health in return. These habits include a healthy diet, focusing on positive healthy food choices: plenty of wholegrains, pulses, fruits, vegetables and oily fish. Keep an eye on your weight and especially your waist (belly fat). Get plenty of exercise. If you smoke cigarettes, stop. Break bad habits. Have a healthy respect for alcohol; while it can be a good servant it is a very bad master. Mind your mental health and watch your stress levels. Don't let what's important to you, including family, friends, hobbies and health, be squeezed too much. Educate and inform yourself about important men's health issues. Have the courage to take control of your own health. Be confident enough to go to the doctor when you feel ill or are concerned about some health issue. Think of your body as being like your car; it too needs its regular NCT.

Prevention Is Better than Cure

You get your car serviced every 20,000 miles, indeed older cars now have to be NCT-tested to ensure their road worthiness. Yet we often fail to apply these minimal basic standards of car welfare to our own bodies and health.

As a family doctor with an interest in men's health I feel that a regular maintenance check or wellness check for men would be a valuable part of every man's health programme. We know that for many reasons men are often 'too busy' to go to the doctor and when they do it is often only after being prodded into action by their partner. So a proper preventative wellness check allows the opportunity and, more importantly, the time to look at the following:

- Your current symptoms, if any
- Your past medical history, including a history of any illnesses and operations, vaccination history, a history of any supplements or over-the-counter vitamins, etc., a history of any allergies, and a critical look at your family history, particularly regarding any potentially inherited diseases such as diabetes, heart disease, bowel cancer, kidney stones and haemochromatosis
- A lifestyle questionnaire, including your exercise habits, diet, alcohol intake and how you deal with stress.
- A physical examination, including body mass index, abdominal circumference, blood pressure, a general examination of your heart, lungs, abdominal area, back and legs, skin surveillance and looking at moles, and an examination of urine
- Make sure you know about any inherited conditions in your family or family illnesses that have a genetic component. There may be specific screening programmes that you can avail of. For example, colonoscopy for polyps, which can lead to bowel cancer, or eye tests to screen for glaucoma (high blood pressure of the eyes). Remember that information and knowledge allow you to make informed decisions for your better health.

As a general rule of thumb I recommend a good check-up for men at the following intervals:

- Every five years for men in their twenties
- Every two to three years for men in their thirties
- Every one to two years for men in their forties
- Over yearly for men in their fifties

Blood tests that may be carried out at these examinations include the following:

- A full blood count – this tests for anaemia (low iron) and the number of white cells (the army that fights infection) in the blood. It also checks the platelet level (the clotting ability of the blood).
- Fasting blood sugar – this tests for diabetes or the likelihood of developing diabetes.
- Lipid profile – this tests the total cholesterol, as well as the LDL (bad) cholesterol, HDL (good) cholesterol and triglyceride (blood fat) levels (see Chapter 6 for a discussion on cholesterol).
- Liver function – this tests the function of the liver.
- Renal function – this checks the kidneys as well as the amount of sodium and potassium in the blood.
- Thyroid – this tests the functioning of the thyroid gland.
- Serum ferritin – this tests the amount of iron stores in the blood.
- Uric acid – this is a screening test for gout.
- PSA – this can be a marker of prostate function (see Chapter 8 for further information on this).

Useful Vaccinations for Men to Consider

- Flu vaccine – recommended annually for men aged over 50 and younger men who have chest problems such as asthma, heart problems, kidney problems, diabetes or a weakened immune system.
- Pneumococcal vaccine – this can provide good protection against the most common type of pneumonia found in the community.
- Hepatitis B vaccine – this protects against the hepatitis B virus, which can be transmitted through body fluids, including via cuts from sports injuries.
- Tetanus vaccine – this protects against tetanus, which can be caused by dirty cuts.

- Travel vaccinations – these are important to remember if you are travelling to other parts of the world.

How To Get the Best from Your Doctor

The following tips may help you get the best from your doctor:

- Treat your doctor as a genuine partner in your healthcare. He or she is there to help you.
- Do not be afraid to ask for help if you are feeling down or stressed.
- Do not be embarrassed asking your doctor about issues you are worried about. He or she is there to help you and has seen and heard it all many times before.
- Do not be afraid to ask questions. The best patient is an informed patient.
- Let your doctor know you are interested in keeping yourself well. Ask about preventative health opportunities, including wellness programmes.
- Consider writing your main symptoms down before you see your doctor. Research has shown that sometimes in consultation we forget to tell or ask our doctor important things that could be bothering us.
- Make sure you understand the benefits and risk of any medication you are prescribed.
- Have a good understanding of your own family history and its relevant health implications. Make sure your doctor does too. Our own individual family history is very important in the context of a risk profile for many health conditions. Do not make assumptions that your doctor knows your father died from bowel cancer twenty years ago. Make sure your doctor is informed of this and that it is recorded prominently in your notes.

- Take some responsibility for the accuracy of your own medical records. Many medical records are now computerised, with specific sections that note drug allergies and past, and family history. Help your doctor to help you by sharing any relevant information.
- Take a balanced approach to any investigations. In the old days time was very important in the context of health, sickness and healing. Time was used both as a diagnostic tool to allow vague symptoms to evolve and as a therapeutic tool to allow symptoms to resolve and nature to take its course. Nowadays, with the advent of medical technology, high-tech scans are often only a fingertip away. While there is no doubt that modern technology has an invaluable role to play in healthcare, over-investigation can cause unnecessary anxiety. Some invasive diagnostic procedures can have risks and side effects of their own but there is a balance here between, on the one hand, the need to evaluate symptoms thoroughly, including appropriate investigation where needed, and, on the other hand, over-investigating everything. With the rise of defensive medicine there can be an extra perceived pressure on your doctor to organise more tests and more scans, so that 'nothing is missed'. Your challenge is to be an informed and equal partner in this decision making. Help your doctor to help you to decide what is best for your long-term health.
- Focus on good communication. Be honest with your doctor and yourself. Learn to talk honestly and openly to your doctor about any worries or concerns you may have. Even if they are of a sensitive nature, your doctor is there to help you. Remember: not even the best doctors can read minds.
- Become proactive and informed on healthcare issues.

- If you are on several medications check out potential drug inter-actions. Make sure you inform your doctor about any supplements or herbal or over-the-counter medications you are taking. This is important because some of these can interact with prescribed medication.
- Stay informed about important developments in men's health.

Why Some Men Do Not Follow Health Advice

Do you know the biggest reason as to why prescribed medication does not work? It is simply because people don't take the medication, or at least don't take enough of it for long enough to produce the desired effect. This is a massive challenge for doctors, patients, healthcare and society in general. There is no doubt that many of us do not like taking pills or medication, particularly if we do not feel sick. I mean, how many of us have been prescribed a week's course of an antibiotic for a sore throat and finished the course? I know many men, doctors included, might take them until they feel better and then stop the rest of the course. While this may not have many adverse consequences for your throat, apart from increasing the risk of drug resistance to antibiotics, the story can be different when you are looking at the management of many chronic conditions, includ-ing high blood pressure, diabetes and high cholesterol. With these conditions, taking medication daily is often essential to maintain wellness and to prevent complications such as heart attack and stroke, which remain among the biggest killers of Irish men.

How Common Is Non-Compliance?

Research has shown that only one in every three men will comply and take a course of medication to a degree sufficient enough to affect outcome. These men, in general, have a better understanding of their medical condition, as well as a better understanding of the need to take medication. Naturally they tend to have better outcomes. About one in three men tend to comply partly with the prescribed medication, in that they may take it for a few months or a year on and off, but not sufficiently frequently enough to prevent complications arising from their condition, and about one in every three men do not comply at all. This lack of compliance does not just apply to pre-scribed medication; it holds for lifestyle advice as well.

There are many reasons as to why Irish men may not comply with healthier advice and prescriptions:

- A man's own health beliefs. We all have our own internal belief systems about health and illness, which are dependent partly on our experiences and upbringing. This is known as the health belief model. Using this model, we all tend to weigh up, on the one hand, our perceived seriousness of the medical condition concerned and how threatened or vulnerable we are to it and, on the other hand, the perceived benefits of doing nothing or of taking action.
- Our level of education is very important. Today, in twenty-first century Ireland, about 15 per cent of Irish men have literacy problems, which act as a huge barrier to informed decision making in the area of health. We are now in the information age where a huge amount of easily accessible evidence-based information is available on a wide range of topics.
- The doctor–patient relationship itself is an integral part of good medical care. You need to trust your doctor, not too much, but enough to allow you to make the best decisions to help yourself in terms of your long-term health and well-being. In the old days, the doctor–patient relationship tended to be quite paternalistic, meaning the doctor assumed the all-knowledgeable father figure role in relation to the subservient child (the

patient). Nowadays, the ideal doctor–patient relationship is thought to be a genuine partnership between you and your doctor. This implies freedom on your part to ask relevant questions, to be heard, to have your ideas, concerns and expectations understood and to be able to discuss things in an open manner. It also gives you the responsibility to act on the shared decisions that you and your doctor come to regarding your health and wellness.

Many people do not comply with medication because they may find it hard to take something several times a day, they may experience side effects, they may have concerns about side effects, potential addiction or dependency, or they may simply find it too expensive. On top of this a man may feel psychologically that his maleness, his manliness, his sense of strength and his invulnerability are threatened by the need to take small pills every day. If you have concerns about any medication prescribed, discuss them with your doctor or pharmacist. I do not think there has ever been a pill made that cannot cause some side effects. Some degree of risk-benefit balancing may have to be done. However, your doctor may be able to suggest more suitable alternatives in many cases.

The Pill-for-every-Ill Culture

If you feel unwell or are concerned about something, you should always see your doctor. However, sometimes the best thing your doctor can prescribe for you is simply good advice. At times the best pill may be no pill at all. For example, many sore throats and upper respiratory infections are caused by viruses, which do not respond to antibiotics and would tend to clear themselves in time, sometimes with the aid of simple over-the-counter remedies. There is evidence that antibiotics are often over-prescribed for sore throats. This can be due to the doctor's perception of the patient's expectation of a prescription, sometimes fuelled by real patient demand for this. So, before you get your next prescription for a sore throat or cough, it might be worth asking the following questions:

- Is this prescription really necessary?
- Can I get better without it?
- What are the benefits of taking this medicine?
- What is the risk of side effects?
- Why am I taking it?
- Are there alternatives?

If you can answer these questions you will have a much better understanding of the need, if any, to take medication. This will help to give you the knowledge, understanding and confidence needed to allow you to comply properly with the treatment given, leading to a better outcome for all.

Making a Change for Your Health

We are all essentially creatures of habit, so making a change is not easy. But making changes by developing newer, healthier habits can be the key to our long-term health and well-being. No matter how unfit you are, no matter how overweight you are, no matter how unhealthy your lifestyle has been up until now, it is never too late to make changes and, in terms of your health, there can be massive benefits just around the corner. I find the following tips useful when looking at positive health changes:

- Write out a balance sheet of all the pluses and minuses to your behaviour change. Get an A4 sheet of paper and draw a line down through the centre. Let's take exercise as an example. On the left-hand side write down all the benefits you will have from taking more exercise. These may include immediate benefits such as feeling better and long-term benefits such as reducing your risk of heart disease and diabetes. On the right-hand side write your perceived negatives for taking more exercise. You should see that one side of the scale (hopefully the left side) far outweighs the other side. This then can act as a tipping point for taking action.

- It can be useful to organise specific strategies to deal with any negatives you may have for making a change. For example, if you feel that lack of time is a negative for taking more exercise then a useful strategy for overcoming this may be to keep an exercise diary over a seven-day period. This will allow you to slot in specific times on certain days for taking exercise. It also provides a useful tool for assessing accurately at the end of each week how much exercise you have taken, which can reinforce the good behaviour. It is important to reward yourself regularly for making a change. Finally, it is important to stay on track; do not get disillusioned or disheartened if you have the occasional slip. We are all human after all. It is what you do 90 per cent of the time that counts for long-term good health.

Challenges Going Forward

There is no doubt that there is an urgent need to advertise and promote men's health in a positive way. Men have been the poor relation in terms of profile, media exposure, funding and lobby groups when it comes to men's health issues. Women have been very proactive in terms of lobbying, quite rightly, for women's health issues, including breast cancer screening and osteoporosis amongst others. These efforts are to be applauded.

However, there has not been the same exposure or drive for important men's health issues, including prostate, bowel and testicular cancer, heart disease, diabetes and depression. The facts of these conditions speak for themselves. Male-specific health strategies must be adopted to try to help those men who haven't been good at helping themselves.

Men's health has a profound impact on all of us in society. It affects the children whose fathers are struck down with premature death or illness and the women whose husbands, fathers, sons and brothers are affected by ill health and premature death. This is not to mention the huge economic and social cost for society. Men's health does indeed reflect the wealth of a nation. It affects all of us. As far as Irish men are concerned, your wealth really is your health. Treasure it!

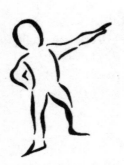

Key Points

- Being an Irish male can be a health hazard.
- Don't let the usual suspects of denial, fear, apathy or 'being too busy' prevent you from taking action.
- Take action and don't become another statistic.
- The gift of better health is within your grasp.
- A healthy lifestyle, including a good diet, exercise and being able to de-stress, is a great way to start the journey to better health.
- Have the same respect for your body and mind as you have for your car – get a regular service.
- Prevention and early detection are better than cure – 'a stitch in time saves nine.'
- Remember that your health is your wealth.

Index